Living with Migraines

Living with Migraines

ALL KINDS OF HEADACHES

G. S. Kathpal, MD

Preface

The main inspiration behind this book was my own headaches, which I have suffered from since the age of eight and still suffer from at the age of sixty-seven, although to a lesser degree. I chose neurology as my specialty because of the complexity of working with the brain, spinal cord, and nerves. I did not choose this specialty to treat my own headaches. The history of headaches is as old as humanity itself. I have described the history of headaches, its understanding and treatment going back more than two centuries. It of course includes the current era of scientific understanding and up-to-date treatment. The origin of headaches, and headaches' symptoms and treatment are in the subsequent chapter. Commonsense treatment and up-to-date modalities have been included. Despite extensive research in the field, only about 40 percent of patients with migraines are properly diagnosed and treated.

Acknowledgments

I would like to thank Vinoo Kathpal for the encouragement, support, and help with research materials. I am also grateful to Colleen Molinaro for her dedication and excellent typing.

Contents

CHAPTER 1

Personal and Family History

I was a little over three years old when my parents fled from Pakistan, where they had lived all their lives. My father worked for the post office when we were transferred to central India.

We lived on the second floor. On the ground floor, there was a Sikh temple, where people came in and out at all times of the day. It got really crowded on Sunday mornings. After a year, my mother got a job as a teacher, and a year after that, she became principal of a new school. She retired from this position at the age of fifty-eight.

There was a physician working on the ground floor of our building. He was very busy and saw almost one hundred patients a day. He was very quick, but he was also a kind person. He did not charge poor patients and would give them free medications. He left a very positive and permanent impression on me.

My father received a couple of promotions, and he was allotted a government bungalow on the outskirts of the city. After we were in this house for two years, he developed a severe attack of eczema (an oozing and itching rash on both feet). He could not go to work for one whole year. He would, however, sign important papers at home. He also took advantage of this time and wrote a book for postal employees. The book was very helpful and sold in every corner of the country.

When I was about eight years old, I was riding my bicycle in the afternoon sun and heat, when at the end of one hour I developed a severe headache in the front of my head. I went home and got sick, and my mother told me to nap. When I woke up after an hour, the headache was gone, and I felt refreshed. Headaches started coming one to two times a month. Some of them responded to naps, but after few months, naps did not help. I was given one tablet of aspirin that did help. After a couple of years, I needed two tablets of aspirins. I developed severe headaches in the front part of my head, which throbbed for a while. Before it subsided, I threw up and then fell asleep. When I woke up after an hour or so, there was no headache, and I felt quite refreshed. Afterward, I asked my parents why I was not taken to see my doctor. They told me it was because both of them got similar headaches and knew what to do. Over the next year or so, the headaches occurred three or four times and responded to naps. When they quit responding to naps, I was given acetaminophen (Tylenol) or aspirin. I found aspirin to be much more effective. These headaches were brought on by exposure to playing in the heat. This was a great tragedy because most sports activities I participated in took place in the sun. The sun shone about three hundred days a year in that part of India. At that point, I learned to swim in a nearby clean river. Then I joined a swim club. Most of the time, I did not get headaches. The trick was to swim for fifteen to twenty minutes and then sit in the shade for some time.

There were two other methods for treating headaches in my family. My father used to do yoga every morning. He informed me that yoga can get rid of headaches for some people. To my horror, every time I did yoga, I got a bad headache—so much for natural treatment. The second method was my own invention. In the mornings when there was enough dew on the grass, I walked barefoot on it if I had a headache. About 80 percent of the time, the headache would go away or at least become much less severe. The problem was that dew appeared on the grass only three months of the year.

From the age of twelve to sixteen years, my headaches became more frequent. They occurred a couple of times a month, with no relief to be had from napping. I now required two, not one, aspirins.

I was always an excellent student and was very competitive. I did very well in most classes and especially in premed. I got into medical school at the age of sixteen. I was very happy to be the youngest in the class. Then I saw the anatomy dissection hall, which contained about thirty naked dead bodies smelling strongly of formaldehyde. To make matters worse, some of the cadavers were missing parts. This scene, along with the thickness of the textbooks, made me think about going to regular college and forgetting about medicine. I also experienced a new kind of headache that I had not anticipated. I started getting headaches at least once a week from the beginning to the end of medical school. Then the headaches came on twice a week. The added bonus was that I was sick 25 percent of the time.

Once I got through the psychological trauma of the first year, things did improve. I scored well in each subject and started out fifth in a class of 150 students. It is worth mentioning that I always got headaches during examinations, and sometimes I needed to ask for a bathroom break. Still, none of this affected my very good scores in the exams. Maybe my resolve was much greater than the stupid migraines.

Throughout medical school I lived on aspirin, sometimes twelve to eighteen a day. They barely took the edge off the pain. I had to buy and hide aspirin at home and keep them in my pocket at work.

Next, I was to face the six-month internship and the three-year residency in internal medicine. The first six months were real murder because I had to work frequent shifts of thirty-six hours. My sleep cycle, of course, was totally disturbed, but my headaches remained the same. Residency was equally vigorous, but there were some brief periods of rest. It was during these three years that the headaches worsened again. These headaches occurred three to four times a week, and they were most severe in the morning. No amount of aspirin would do any good, and it irritated my stomach. At that time, there was a pill called Saridon (composed of aspirin, salicylic acid, caffeine, and a small amount of codeine). I tried just one, and it worked wonderfully. I depended on these pills for three years. Sometimes I had to take two, though. My mother used to take the same pills with good results, but she never told me about them. When I confronted her, she said once she started taking Saridon, nothing else worked, and that was the reason she did not tell me.

My Father

My father had headaches on both sides of his head beginning at the age of seventeen. They remained infrequent, occurring only once or twice a month, and then they occurred three to four times a week.

As I observed him over many years, he had two types of headaches. One was the garden-variety migraine without aura. He usually woke up with these, but sometimes they occurred at the end of the day. Pain was on one side, with the throbbing lasting for several hours to all day. Sometimes, the migraine was associated with nausea, vomiting, excessive urination, and diarrhea. He was wary of medications and would depend on plain aspirin. He finally found a neurologist who was trained in the United States. He made the right diagnosis of migraine headaches and asked my father to take one tablet of Cafergot (ergotamine and caffeine) at the onset of a headache. It worked well as long as he could keep the pill in his stomach. Vomiting was an issue with 25 percent of his headaches. I suggested that he take something for nausea and wait for thirty minutes before taking Cafergot. This also worked. At the age of about forty, he started getting cluster headaches. These are described later in chapter 10.

By the time he got to age fifty-five, his headaches started to become less severe and less frequent. His headaches went away at the age of seventy years.

Much has been written about the personalities of people who suffer from migraines. These sufferers are compulsive and perfectionists, have a high incidence of anxiety and depression, and find it difficult to accept defeat. My father was a pleasant person who was neither compulsive at home or at work, although he did take his work very seriously.

My Mother

She started getting migraines and menstrual headaches since she was about twenty-five years old. Her worst headaches were on the first day of her menstrual cycle. She invariably got sick and needed injectable medicine to control nausea. She responded to Saridon most of the time. Sometimes, she needed an injection for pain. She continued to get a mild headache every day and took one or two Saridons a day until she passed away at the age of eighty-nine years. She was an aggressive high achiever and had frequent mood swings. She was also a perfectionist. She fitted the mold of migraine personality.

My Brother

He had his first migraine at the age of twenty-three. In general, his headaches are less frequent and less severe than my father and me.

My father does not recall anyone having headaches in his immediate family. There are ten siblings in my mother's family. Five of them had a significant degree of migraine headaches. There are many other members of the family who get migraines. These include my brother's son, too.

My Daughters

I have two daughters. The older had her first migraine while she was playing on the beach in the sun. She was four years old. My daughters had headaches while playing tennis in the sun. Giving them Motrin thirty minutes before playing time could prevent that. The older daughter had headaches in her late teens and early twenties. She responded well to Nadalol for prevention and Sumatriptan for the headache. Now, she rarely gets headaches. My younger daughter does not get any headaches.

My Wife

I got married in India to an Indian girl in September 1971. In 1973, we had a healthy and beautiful baby girl.

My wife of course is not my blood relative but started having mostly menstrual headaches at the age of thirty-four years. I tried her on ten different medications, and the tenth one worked. A medicine called Sansert worked for her for almost twenty years. Late in the 1950s, scientists were working on serotonin. A drug was developed by the name of Sansert, which works by serotonin-like action and to some degree by anti-serotonin like action. Now, she gets occasional headaches, which respond to Motrin. Her father used to get headaches, too.

My residency in internal medicine was coming to an end. I appeared in the boards of internal medicine and stood first in the university. I had two choices: one was to go into private practice of internal medicine in the same town; the other was to specialize in some other branch of medicine. In the late 1960s, there were very few treatments for neurological diseases. The part that was most stimulating was the mental aspect. Once a diagnosis or possible diagnosis was made, not a whole lot could be done for 90 percent of the patients.

I applied for the job of registrar in neurology at the All India Institute of Medical Sciences. It was, and still is, the best medical school, research institute, and hospital located in New Delhi. I was the only candidate chosen for the job—they even rejected their own candidates. It was a great place to learn. It was the referral center for the northern and central parts of the country. I was amazed by the variety of both common and very uncommon diseases I encountered—many of which I had not seen before and probably will not see again.

I was seriously considering going to the United States, which required an entrance exam. The Indian government stopped giving these exams because it did not want any trained doctors to leave the country. In 1971, I went to Iran to pass the entrance examination (ECFMG) to get a residency in America. I applied to seven universities and was offered jobs by three of them.

I had a very modest exposure to drugs. I was always afraid to take street drugs because of the safety factor. I did try the stimulant Ritalin, mostly to stay up all night. I was able to read all night, but I was not sure if I would remember everything I had studied. I soon gave up on that idea.

In July 1972, I joined a residency program in the northeastern United States. I was hoping it would last less than three years, but that did not work out. I showed up for a Saturday morning meeting. The chairman introduced me to everyone and talked with me for a few minutes.

The chairman of neurology was less than forty years old, energetic, and extremely knowledgeable, including having good general knowledge. He was an excellent teacher and was tireless. Now, I was going to get some real training in neurology.

I was running out of my pain pills, so I asked the chairman if he could write me a couple of tablets. He refused to give me the preventive medicine Sansert, saying it was risky. He put me on another medicine called Bellergal Space-tabs (composed of ergotamine, caffeine, belladonna, and aspirin), whose dosage was twice a day. It did not work, so he increased it to two tablets twice a day. He also gave me a prescription for a pain medication called Fiorinal (aspirin, barbiturates, and caffeine); he said that the thirty tablets should last a month or so. I did not know if I should laugh or cry, but I did not want to argue with him. His secretary, who was listening to the conversation, told me later that she would get me a bottle of one hundred from one of the drug representatives. In six months, I got my license, and I could write my own prescriptions.

The first year of my residency was getting close. I had always wanted to work at Massachusetts General Hospital at Harvard University in Boston. I was granted permission for an interview. They offered me a position but starting as a first-year resident, which I found totally unacceptable. Then I came back to talk to my chairman to see if it was possible to reduce my residency to two years. He was very well aware that I had spent endless years in training. He told me, rather candidly, that he could do that, but it would be very difficult to appear for neurology boards, which meant I would not be getting too many positions in this country. However, he made me an offer that was hard to refuse. He offered me the job of assistant professor at the university the next day after finishing my training. He did not need the answer right away. With all the thoughts running through my head, I forgot to ask what he was going to pay me.

The Bellergal Space-tabs were beginning to become less effective. There was now a new class of drugs called beta-blockers. There was a patient in a hospital in Miami who had heart disease. He also had a history of lifelong migraines. The first of these drugs, called propranolol (Inderal), was given to him. Surprisingly, not only did his heart condition improve, but his migraines went away as well. I took the pill as soon as I could lay my hands on it. To my big disappointment, I was allergic to it. I had to wait for a year before a second pill in the same category came by. The name of the new pill was Noradol (Corgard), and I was able to take that without any difficulty. I started with a tablet of 80 mg once a day and gradually increased it to three a day. In about three weeks, there was substantial improvement. I quit taking Bellergal Space-tabs but did use the Fiorinal as needed.

When I was about thirty years old and my wife and I were making love, I had a sudden burst of pain in the back of my head and neck; the pain lasted for an hour. I did take some Fiorinal as soon as I could. Still, it was difficult to understand why an act so pleasurable could be associated with so much pain. I did study this condition and found few medicines that could help the situation. Taking a tablet of Cafergot or 25–50 mg of indomethacin (Indocin; a nonsteroidal anti-inflammatory drug) could help immediately. I was still mad because it was not the first time, nor would it be the last. I tried both of the medications one at a time, and Cafergot seemed to work much better.

The first year of residency was a highly rewarding experience, and I was looking forward to the other two years. My chairman was very sensitive to my needs—not that I was handicapped in any way. The things he paid special attention to were the US versions of British words or phrases. I knew most of them anyway, but I would let him go on. He used spatula instead of tongue blade, flashlight instead of torch, and so on. Once I was presented with a patient who I thought was white but was in fact black. Later on, the chairman took me to that patient's room and showed me all the reasons why he was a black man. He also gave me tips on how to avoid medical malpractice cases. One of the other things he tried to teach me was abuse and proper use of painkillers, especially narcotics.

The next two years of residency were as fruitful as the first. I wrote scientific papers under the guidance of three different staff members.

As was decided before, I was appointed assistant professor of neurology. This required me to see patients in private doctors' offices independently and to teach medical students, interns, medical residents, psychiatry residents, and neurology and neurosurgery residents. I'd had enough experience in this matter in the past that I could do it with ease and effectiveness. My students wanted me to teach them all the time instead of other staff members.

The chairman liked to give lectures to medical students all the time because he thought he could do the best job of it. After about six months, he asked me to give a lecture to the medical students. He told me he would take out the slides and make them available, along with appropriate literature. I made one request to him, which was that he should not come to the lecture theater where I was giving the talk. I also told him I would take care of everything, and I would ask for help only if needed. I felt that his biggest concern was if the students would be able to understand me. I still had a slight accent but not as heavy as it had been three and a half years before. Soon after the lecture began, a bunch of neurology residents as well as medical students slowly infiltrated the room and occupied the empty seats, especially in the back row. I felt I was doing a good job. The long and loud standing ovation at the end of my lecture confirmed my belief. The chairman kept his promise and was waiting in his office two floors below. He did not need any confirmation and was very pleased. He told me I could give lectures at any time.

There is one patient during my time in a private office who I find difficult to forget. The patient was about twenty-five years old with a history of chronic headaches. He described them as extremely bad and occurring almost continuously. After I took his history and asked him to take off some of his clothes, I saw that he had three bullet wounds. I had never seen bullet wounds before. I asked him what they were about, and he told me that one was from Cleveland, the other from Detroit, and the third from New York. He basically wanted a hundred tablets of Percodan. I told him I simply could not do that. I wanted to run some tests before deciding what kind of medications he needed. I wrote a prescription for twenty tablets of Percodan. He got extremely loud and mad, tore up the prescription, and threw it on the floor. He also threatened me by saying that when I came down the escalator at noon the next day; he was going to shoot me with a 45-caliber revolver. In addition, he left several messages with the secretary of the neurology office. I knew intuitively that people who threaten like this usually don't kill; it's the psychotic, silent types who are more likely to do that. I stayed home for one day and came back to work the following day. I had called the police, who told me "unless he takes a shot at you, we cannot do anything about it." Fifteen years later, I got a message on my beeper—we did not have cell phones in those days—and I answered the call. There was a familiar voice on the other end, and he told me he needed fifty tablets of Percodan. I told him I did not have a prescription pad in my car or on my person, but if he came the next day, I would be happy to see what I could do. He simply hung up. About two months later, he was killed in a drug deal.

Things changed at the university. The chairman resigned from his chair but stayed on as a full professor. He continued to support me in every way possible, but still, it changed my future.

There were two techniques on the horizon: one was a CAT (computerized axial tomography) scan, which showed very clear slices of the brain, spinal cord, and discs. The diagnoses that could only be surmised in the past could now be diagnosed with authority. I'd never thought such a day would come. The second technique was the evoked response test (now called evoked potential test). It consisted of three parts: visual, brain stem, and somatosensory-evoked responses. When one stimulated the eyes, ears, or nerves of the arms and legs, small-amplitude responses were magnified by repeated stimulation. This test was most useful in patients with multiple sclerosis but could also be used in other situations. Spinal taps were used frequently in various neurological conditions including possible multiple sclerosis; however, with the evoked response test, one could avoid the spinal tap, which is a painful procedure and consists of insertion of a needle in between two vertebrae to obtain spinal fluid for analysis.

We had a new chairman from Miami, who brought about ten staff members with him. The work was drastically reduced for everyone. I saw patients in private offices only once a week but made rounds with the residents twice a week. Some days, there was nothing to do at all. I absolutely hated that. One could only read so much during the day.

I talked with the new chairman about the possibility of doing a three-month fellowship to learn the technique of evoked responses. I opted to go to San Diego.

After I came back from my fellowship, I talked with the new chairman about the possibility of buying the equipment for evoked response testing. The cost was approximately $24,000; this cost would be recovered in a year's time. I talked with him on three or four other occasions, but he had deaf ears each time.

Consequently, I decided to open a lab and got two more investors, including my old chairman to purchase the equipment. Because it was the first in town, we got a lot of referrals from hundreds of miles away. The cost was recouped in the first year as predicted. The old chairman was very eager to read the tests, but he didn't know how. One day, he came to me and asked me if I could teach him this. He came with a bunch of papers and took notes very diligently. I thought to myself that that was the first time I would teach him something when in the past, it was he who had imparted so much knowledge to me.

The new chairman was furious about this private lab. He went running to the dean's office to see if I could be fired. I thought my contract was for three years, but in fact it was for six years. The only person who knew about it was my old chairman.

I tried to increase my dosage of Corgard to four tablets because that was pretty much all I could take. The headaches were not as well controlled as they had been before. At this juncture, still another class of medications came on the market called calcium channel blockers. They were heart medications, but they also prevented the blood vessels from enlarging and throbbing, which helped with migraines. The first calcium channel blocker was verapamil, and I tried a dose of 200 mg once a day. It did help to a moderate degree. I put myself back on two tablets of Corgard, and that combination worked well. In fact, I continued to take this combination for twelve years. Eventually, I had to increase the Corgard and surprisingly was able to take eight to ten tablets of Corgard 80 mg daily. I had to check my blood pressure from time to time, but there were no other problems.

In 1977, we had another healthy baby girl. My wife wanted to have a son, but what could we do? Both times my wife was pregnant, I picked only girls' names, which irritated her even more.

I stayed at the university until the summer of 1981. I joined a suburban practice with a colleague who was one year senior to me in residency. I was ready for a change because there was just too much time at hand. The work was somewhat hard but interesting and monetarily rewarding. I worked with him for thirteen years.

After the CAT scan, there was a newer scan called magnetic resonance imaging (MRI). Here, a powerful magnet was used to produce
images. It was much more sensitive compared to the CAT scan and could
show rather small areas of anomaly.

I had gall bladder surgery in 1986. The postoperative period was
very painful. I was kept in the hospital for fourteen days. I got Demerol
injections around the clock while I was in the hospital. I did not have
any headaches during those two weeks. This is a well-known phenom-
enon: after general anesthesia, headaches go away for seven to ten days.
Second, when the mind is occupied with pain in another part of the
body, it somehow takes over, and you don't feel the pain. I was hoping
the headaches would not visit me again, but no such luck. If my headache
was moderate, I would use the pills I was taking, but if the headache was
extremely painful, I would take an injection. I used the injections rather
sparingly. Initially, it was only a few times a month, but that frequency
became once a week, and then two to three times a week. I tapered and
discontinued the injection over a period of one week.

I split with my partner and opened the first headache center in the
city. I saw about 75 percent headache patients and 25 percent other neurological patients. Things got busy rather quickly.

There was another exciting development in the area of headache
treatment. Glaxo in England spent ten years and a billion dollars and
came up with a product called Imitrex (sumatriptan), which has properties related to serotonin. First, it came in the form of an injection and
then in tablets. I took an injection when my headache was full blown.
The nausea and headache went away within thirty minutes or so. I did
not have any side effects. I gave injections to many patients with very en-
couraging results. Some patients had side effects in the form of tingling
in the head, dizziness, chest pain, and rapid heartbeat. Side effects went
away in ten to fifteen minutes. About 70 percent of patients who could
tolerate the injections did well with them. When the tablet form came
out about six months later, I had excellent response to it, too. Roughly
66 percent of patients also did very well. Side effects were very few.

In the fall of 1991, I woke up at 4:00 a.m. with a severe pain, like a
poker going through my head. I could not stay in bed and paced the
room most of the time. The pain was intense and devastating but not

throbbing. The pain was on my right side in the front area of my head and behind my eye. My right eye was shut, and that eye and the right side of my nose were watering. Thanks to that new injection of Imitrex, my pain was gone in about twenty minutes. This occurred at 4:00 a.m. every day for a few days and sometimes occurred ninety minutes after I went to sleep. All other symptoms and signs were the same. These lasted for three consecutive nights. This reminded me of the kind of very similar headaches my father used to get. I was hoping that the migraines were bad enough and somehow I would skip the cluster headaches. The headaches were more tolerable because of these new injections.

I had a bad automobile accident in January 1992. My headaches disappeared soon after the accident, but after about two months, they returned with a vengeance. The preventive medicines that had helped me for so long quit working. I wanted to start myself on a very old antidepressant by the name of phenelzine (Nardil). It had so many restrictions of food and medications that I wanted to get a second opinion. I went to see the head of the headache department at the Cleveland Clinic. I did know him to some extent. We agreed that I could start phenelzine. The dose was three to four tablets a day. Over a period of six days, I was at the full dose. By the fifth or sixth day, the headaches went away completely.

The medication worked for me for seven to eight years and then quit. I tried to give up phenelzine on three different occasions. I cut one quarter of a pill every three weeks, but when I got down to three pills, the headaches became much more intense. The same thing happened all three times. I left myself on phenelzine as before and added something safe. I was not getting the intense migraine type of headaches but had a dull and diffuse pain every day.

After Imitrex came on the market, two other triptans, zolmitriptan (Zomig) and rizatriptan (Maxalt), appeared. They were very similar. In my estimation, Imitrex was the most potent. However, different patients responded well to one medicine or another. Unfortunately, they were all very expensive at fifteen to twenty dollars a pill. The insurance company would give six pills a month. For most patients, it was just not enough. Despite this great medicine, we still had to write prescriptions for tablets like Vicodin and Fiorinal. Finally, there were four more pills introduced, so there was a better choice.

About three years after I started phenelzine (Nardil), I developed symptoms of hypomania (a lesser form of mania). I slept very poorly, talked a lot, frequently went shopping for things I did not need, and became easily irritable and angry. This was the total opposite of my personality. I was usually quiet and spoke when necessary, was soft spoken, and was congenial. I realized that this was due to phenelzine. I talked to my headache physician, and he agreed that this was probably from phenelzine. He recommended that I change my dosage. After a couple of years, I developed similar symptoms on three pills of phenelzine. He decided to stop the medication altogether and tried a new medication. The name of the new medication was protriptyline (Vivactil), which was another antidepressant. I started taking three pills a day. There was some confusion as to how to switch the medications. My impression was that I needed to stop phenelzine for two weeks and then start Vivactil. My doctor suggested that I drop one tablet of phenelzine and add one tablet of Vivactil. This needed to be done every five days or so. I was not too pleased with this method, but I thought he was more experienced in those matters. I did not develop any side effects at the time.

The side effects of phenelzine and Vivactil were very much alike; they consisted of poor sleep, poor appetite and pressure of speech (meaning talking relentlessly without making too much sense), unusual laughing, and use of vulgar language at times. I also had some degree of hallucinations, poor reasoning, loss of memory, and loss of concentration. Manic-depressive illness has an incidence of familial disease, but in my case, I could not find anyone who had that.

I stopped Vivactil because that turned out to be the culprit. I was also put on lithium 300 mg three times a day and Thorazine (an antipsychotic medication) 25mg two times a day.

Once I stopped Vivactil and phenelzine, after about three weeks the headaches came back. I again started phenelzine but with no benefit. The first antiepileptic drug I tried was about fifteen years old, and its name was Depakote (valproate). I started on a dose of 500mg two times a day. I had some abdominal pain and diarrhea. These symptoms disappeared in three weeks. In about a month, the headaches improved. I could take Depakote with other medications. Unfortunately, at the end of three months, I had gained fifteen pounds, so I had to stop the Depakote.

The next drug I tried was tiagabine (Gabitril), and the dose was slowly increased to 1,000mg a day. There were very few side effects. I had about 60 percent improvement in the headaches at the end of one month, but that was just not enough. Next, I tried Neurontin (gabapentin) on a dose that was gradually increased to 1,800mg per day. At the end of one month, I had absolutely no improvement.

Next came Topamax in the year 2000. The dose was started at 25mg a day and increased to 100mg a day. The side effects were dizziness, sleepiness, and weight loss. I had no trouble taking the medicine. At the end of one month, there was 80 percent improvement. Unfortunately, after a year, the medicine quit working altogether.

What followed was another antiepileptic medication, lamotrigine (Lamictal), which was an excellent antiepileptic drug with few side effects. It was proven that it was 68 percent effective in the prevention of migraine headaches. However, for me, the result was 0 percent.

The next drug I tried was levetiracetam (**Keppra**). The side effects included excessive sleepiness, irritation, tiredness, and psychosis. It was quite effective, at 74 percent in most patients. I could not tolerate this medication, though.

Next was tiagabine (**Gabitril**), which worked like Topamax. Its side effects were sleepiness, dizziness, and fatigue. In several of the studies, it worked in about 60 percent of the patients in the prevention of migraines. I had no benefit from this medicine either.

The last anticonvulsant was zonisamide (Zonegran). The side effects included tingling, fatigue, anxiety, and weight loss. The dose was 400 mg a day. In multiple studies, it was reported to be effective in 50 to 65 percent of patients with migraines. This medicine did help me for some time.

CHAPTER 2

Historical Review

M any famous people from the past had migraines including Thomas Jefferson, John Calvin, Albert Einstein, Mary Tudor, Adolf Hitler, Jesus Christ, Lee Grant, Immanuel Kant, Edgar Allan Poe, Julius Caesar, Charles Darwin, Peter Tchaikovsky, Leo Tolstoy, Harold Wolff, Blaise Pascal, Lewis Carroll, Friedrich Nietzsche, Saint Paul, Frederic Chopin, Karl Marx, Alfred Nobel, Sigmund Freud, and Queen Elizabeth II's sister, Princess Margaret.

History of Migraines Continued

Humankind has had headaches since the dawn of civilization. In the seventh century, Ninivech described various severe internal diseases including headaches. It would not be wrong to interpret that flashing lightning, which he described as like a star of fire full of cloud, as a migraine aura. One of the explanations was that demons caused this. These headaches were treated with a variety of animals tied to one side of the head. An Egyptian book of medicine written between 1500 bce and 250 ce has been translated as describing a migraine, but it mentions a one-sided headache without the other features of a migraine, which might well be a cluster headache, trigeminal neuralgia, dental infection, or infestation as a result of cancer.

Trephining of the skull (opening of a hole in the skull) was one of the treatments the Egyptians used for a long time. They believed this got rid of poisonous or noxious fumes, letting them out of the body.

In Rome in the first century ce, the great physician Aretaeus of Cappadocia wrote a book on neurology, which included headaches, epilepsy, and hysteria. In the second century ce, Galen of Pergamum, another Greek doctor in Rome, stipulated that a migraine is caused by yellow bile irritating intracranial structures. However, the noxious mantle is held back by the falx cerebri (a tough fibrous tissue that keeps the two sides of the brain apart). According to him, throbbing pain originates from blood vessels. Some of it comes from the nerves. Galen's idea of yellow bile from the liver causing migraines came from some of his colleagues in France, where some people still believe such ideas to this day.

Finally, the International Headache Society developed a real scientific classification in 1988, where the differentiation of migraines from tension-type headaches was pivotal.

Migraines and Other Headaches: A Patient's Perspective

There are many kinds of headaches besides migraines. Even though migraines will be covered in great detail in this book, other kinds of headaches will be considered as well.

Finally, the important aspects of causation of headaches, the investigation needed, the prophylactic and preventive medication and acute treatment, and the roles of diet, sleep, food, exercise, smoking, and alcohol are considered in chapter 3.

It is estimated that roughly eighty million people suffer from migraines. Estimates of lifetime prevalence range from 8 to 29 percent for adult females and 4 to 19 percent for adult males. The incidence of migraines is approximately four times more common in women than in men.

Headache is one of the most frequently reported symptoms in the adult general population, which makes it even more common than the common cold. In France, the reported prevalence is 11.9 percent for women and 4.0 percent for men. Similar numbers exist for other European countries. Four percent of the population seeks medical attention for headaches. It is also estimated that almost everyone will have one headache each year. Epidemiology studies compare some of the Western countries as far as these headaches are concerned. Roughly 2 percent of the population of Nigeria and Zimbabwe has been reported to have migraines. The incidence in India is roughly 2 percent, and the incidence in China is 1 percent. This incidence may be related to poor data collection, poor symptom communication, diet, a more laid-back life, and so on.

Incidence of Migraines in Various Countries

Country	Percentage
Turkey	24.7
India	2
France	5
Denmark	18
Sweden	14
United States	12
Germany	27
Croatia	19
Italy	12
Saudi Arabia	2.6
China	0.63
Hong Kong	1.5
Japan	8.5
Malaysia	9
Taiwan	9.1
Ethiopia	3
Korea	22.3

Differences in geography, culture, genetics, ethnicity, and food probably affect this kind of difference in incidence of migraines in different countries.

CHAPTER 3

Genetics and Scientific Basis of Headaches

By and large, headaches are an inherited disorder in 80 to 90 percent of patients. Transmission of migraines from parent to child was noted in the seventeenth century. Tissot first noted the familial aggregation of migraines in 1790. Chromosome 12 was demonstrated to be responsible for transmission of familial hemiplegic migraines, when a person gets weakness on one side of the body and gets headache on the other side of the body. If one person has migraines, half of his or her offspring will also have migraines. If both parents have migraines, chances are that 100 percent of their children will have migraines. Chromosomes 19 and 1 are responsible for the transmission of migraines with and without aura. Incidence in mono- and dizygotic twins is almost similar.

The mode of inheritance can be X-linked (mother to child) or autosomal dominant or recessive, which can come from either parent. If one parent has migraine 50% of children will have migraines and if both parents have migraines all the children will have migraines.

Serotonin is involved in the causation of migraines. In association analyses, no significant difference was found in migraine without aura in the general population. A Danish-Scottish study found that the rate of allelic relay of the human ion transport gene is susceptible to migraines.

Nitrous oxide has been implicated in the causation of migraines.

Individuals with migraines with auras have significantly increased frequencies of dopamine D2 receptor genes.

Cause of Headaches

The exact cause of headaches is a matter of conjecture. Headaches can be divided into primary headaches, in which symptoms and disease processes are unknown, and secondary headaches, in which headaches are symptoms of some other disease or illness. Migraines are a paroxysmal (episodic or occurring from time to time) disease. Involvement of large intracranial vessels, dura mater, and trigeminal systems causes pain on one side of the head. The dura mater is the outermost covering of the brain. The trigeminal nerve carries sensations from one half of the head to opposite side of brain.

The structures that perceive pain include large intracranial vessels, pial vessels (in the covering of the brain), large venous sinuses, and dura mater. The trigeminal fibers innervate the central vessels from the nerves to the trigeminal ganglion. Pain is processed in the thalamus (a large cell mass in the middle and sometimes part of the occipital cortex).

The nucleus (the cluster of cells in the upper brain stem) is the part of the brain that connects the spinal cord to the cerebral hemisphere (two halves of the brain). Electrodes planted in this area for relief of pain can cause migraines. This theory rules that not only the structures just outlined are responsible for pain, but also the brain itself is also capable of perceiving pain. This theory rules out the long-standing one that suggests the brain did not feel pain.[1]

In some ways, there is validation of the widening of intracranial arteries as well as coverings of the brain, pial, and dural coverings. These are often brought on by exposure to heat, sun, different chemicals, emotional factors, and so forth. This, in turn, causes exudation (leaking out of the blood vessels) of certain chemicals and neurotransmitters (chemical messengers in the brain that take information from one part of the brain to the other). The chemical inflammation locates in the blood vessels. Finally, pain impulses are transmitted to the thalamus, cerebral cortex, and trigeminal nerve.

---

1 Neil Raskin, "Cause of Pain," in *Headache*, 2nd ed. (New York: Churchill Livingston, 1988).

It can be said without much reservation that the exact cause of migraines is still unknown. However, research in the past sixty years and especially in the last twenty-five years has shed considerable light on this matter.

Pain-Sensitive Structures in the Head

The veins and arteries in the brain, large venous sinuses, and dura at the base of the brain are pain-sensitive structures. It was maintained for a long time that the brain is insensitive to pain.

Dr. Neil Raskin studied fifteen patients with no prior history of migraines. Electrodes were implanted in the thalamus and part of the brain stem for chronic back pain. Thirteen out of fifteen patients developed migraine-type headaches. This is a strong argument in favor of the brain being capable of producing pain.

Blood vessels in the brain are supplied by nerves with several chemicals (neurotransmitters), such as norepinephrine, acetylcholine, serotonin (5HT), and substance P. These act as chemical messengers.

Acceptable Blood-Flow Studies

Pressure applied to or compression of the carotid artery on the side of the migraine reduces the intensity of the headache. When ergotamine is given to a patient who is having a migraine, it reduces the intensity of the migraine as well as the pulsatile force.

Migraine with Aura

First, there is decreased circulation in the area of the brain that causes aura. This is followed in three to six hours by increased circulation, which causes clinical manifestation.

Serotonin

This is one of the most common messengers in the brain. It has been studied since the 1950s. Many of the medications developed since then have been serotonin-type medications. It is generally the migraine population that has a reduced amount of serotonin in the upper brain stem.

In conclusion, migraines are a hereditary disease with paroxysmal pulsatile pain on one side of the head and are usually associated with nausea,

Vomiting, sensitivity to light, and sensitivity to sound, with some patients having brief periods of neurological deficits such as loss of vision, dizziness, numbness, and weakness on one side of the body. There is an inborn deficiency of serotonin in the upper brain stem.

Medical Conditions Associated with Migraines

Certain medical conditions occur with migraines in a large proportion of patients:

Strokes	4% of patients
Low blood pressure	20% of patients
Ulcers	22% of patients
Heart attacks	11% of patients
Epilepsy	2.1% of patients
Allergies	35% of patients
Angina	8% of patients
Asthma	24% of patients
Colitis	9% of patients
Anxiety	3% of patients
Depression	3.5% of patients

Causes and tests for migraines

Blood-Flow Changes in Migraines

First, there is decreased blood flow in the occipital lobe-both parts of the head in the back, which is responsible for auras of vision. This is followed by a period of increased perfusion of circulation, which generally has no clinical correlation (no symptoms).

Immunological Diseases in Headaches

There is a high incidence of rheumatoid arthritis, lupus (systemic lupus erythematosus), and lichen planus (chronic inflammatory skin rash in the neck, axilla, and groin).

EEG (Electroencephalogram)

This is a study of the electrical activity of the brain. This can be compared to EKG (electrocardiogram) for the study of heart rhythms. EEG changes when a person is having a migraine; it shows a high degree of slow activity. Sometimes, there is increased sharp activity. Patients not having migraines tend to have a somewhat higher percentage of abnormality but mostly slow activity. EEG is not a very good tool for making a diagnosis; it is most valuable in making a diagnosis of epilepsy, which sometimes occurs with migraine headaches.

Nitrous Oxide in Migraines

Nitrous oxide is present in the brain, endothelium (innermost lining of vessels), heart, and so forth. Hormones and chocolate tend to increase nitrous oxide directly or indirectly. Some of the new drugs that have been tried are related to the action of nitrous oxide.

Discriptions of Migraines

Migraines without Aura

These are recurring headaches lasting four to seventy-two hours. They are unilateral, throbbing, and moderate to severe in intensity with nausea; cause sensitivity to light and sound; and are aggravated by physical activity. They are also called atypical or common migraine headaches.

Premonitory Symptoms

Premonitory symptoms last one or two days and include physical or mental hyper- or hypo-activity, depression, craving for foods, excessive sleep, and so on.

Aura

Most common are visual auras such as loss of vision, zigzag lines in front of the eyes, partial loss of vision, numbness or weakness on one or both sides of the body, and loss of balance. The duration of these can be thirty minutes to forty-eight hours.

Headache

Usually the headache is on one side and in the frontal area of the head behind the eyes, temporal areas, and sometimes the back of the head. Associated symptoms such as nausea, vomiting, sensitivity to light and sound, perspiration, fainting, and confusion can occur.

Frequency of Attacks

These can be one per year to three or four attacks per week. Attacks are more frequent in migraines without aura.

Resolution of Attacks

Attacks fade away slowly after the person sleeps for a few hours. Symptoms of nausea or vomiting also sometimes resolve the attacks. Several symptoms occur during the recovery phase; these are change in mood, muscle weakness, tiredness, and feeling washed out and mentally below par. On average, these symptoms last for about twenty-four hours.

Other Types of Migraines without Aura

Menstrual Migraines

These headaches can last from two days before the menstrual cycle up to a couple of days after the menstrual cycle. They can involve headache in between menstrual cycles as well. The majority of sufferers have migraines without auras, but some do have auras and other associated symptoms such as nausea and vomiting.

Status Migrainosus

Here, the migraine lasts for seventy-two to ninety-six hours. It starts as a migraine and then develops features of tension-type headaches. These attacks are also very difficult to treat. The exact cause of this is not very well understood. Swelling of the brain and increased circulation in the brain are incomplete explanations. Emotional distress, depression, anxiety, and abuse of medications, especially ergotamine, are possible explanations.

Migraines with Aura

Auras are neurological deficits developing over a period of five to twenty minutes and usually lasting up to an hour. Headaches and associated symptoms usually occur after the aura is over. Sometimes, there is only an aura but no headache. Headaches usually last from four to ninety-six hours.

Visual Auras

These are the most common auras and present in many forms:

Fortification—Objects appear surrounded by colorful angels that are enlarged, hence the word *fortified*

Zigzag lines

Scintillating scotomas—the vision gets brighter and then dimmer, Loss of vision in both eyes. Loss of vision on one side or loss of a quarter of vision, and so fort

Sensory Aura This consists of tingling and loss of sensation in one extremity, two extremities, or all four extremities; sensory symptoms of the face; and so forth. These symptoms can last for one to seven days.

Motor Aura—Symptoms include weakness in one arm, one arm and one leg, all four extremities, and face with one arm. Motor auras have similar duration as sensory auras.

Language Aura—Disturbance or difficulty in understanding speech, being unable to speak, and slow speech are seen in this particular aura. These are, however, much less frequent.

Symptoms That Are Not Necessarily Auras

Such symptoms include dizziness, decreased level of consciousness, low blood pressure, low heart rate, syncope (loss of consciousness upon standing up), nausea, vomiting, and confusion. These are not necessarily part of auras but can be part of migraine headaches.

CHAPTER 4

Classification of Headaches

Differential Diagnosis of Headaches
Primary headaches
Migraines with aura
Migraines without aura
Ophthalmoplegic headaches—visual symptoms with headaches
Retinal migraines—loss of vision without headaches
Childhood vertigo of intermittent type—this condition usually occurs
    in families in which other members have had migraine headaches.
    Children from age four to ten develop dizziness that is intermittent
    and often associated with abdominal pain and vomiting.
Periodic abdominal pain—this condition also occurs in children when
    some other members in their family have had migraines. They get
    intermittent attacks of abdominal pain but not necessarily dizziness
    and headaches.

Tension-type headaches
Cluster headaches
Episodic—occurring from time to time
Chronic—occurring for months to years at a time
Chronic paroxysmal hemicranias—this involves severe, jabbing pain
    on one side of the head and is usually well treated with one of

the arthritis-type pills called Indocin; this can also be treated with Cafergot.

Other headaches

Cold-stimulus headaches—these are brought on by eating ice cream too fast and usually occur in children. These headaches last for only about twenty minutes, sometimes half an hour. However, sometimes the pain can last a couple of hours if not treated.

Stabbing headaches—these headaches stab on both sides of the head, and their intensity of pain is a little less than chronic paroxysmal hemicranias.

Benign cough headaches—patients with a history of chronic lung disease, if they have a bad bout of coughing, sometimes develop a throbbing pain in their heads, most of the time in the occipital regions.

Benign exertional headaches—these are brought on by any kind of exercise; most of the time, they are brought on by unaccustomed exercise such as playing tennis, lifting weights, or any other physical activity. These headaches can be treated prophylactically by one of the arthritis pills such as Motrin, Indocin, or Cafergot, to be taken half an hour before exercise.

Headaches brought on by sexual activity—patients with migraine headaches sometimes get intense headaches right before coitus, and it does not have anything to do with the intensity of the physical exertion. These can also be treated by some prophylactic medications as mentioned above.

Secondary headaches

Where the cause is know

Head trauma

Associated with vascular disorders

Acute stroke

Bleeding in the head

Subarachnoid bleed- Bleeding between two layers of the coating of the brain. The rupture of an aneurysm often brings this on, which is a weak area on the blood vessel that forms into a balloon.

Arthritis—inflammation in and outside of the head in the blood vessels

High blood pressure—most of the time, a mild to moderate amount of high blood pressure does not cause headaches. However, if blood pressure is extremely high, in the range of 180–240 systolic and 100–130 diastolic, headaches can occur.

Other intracranial disorders

Acute stroke

Bleeding in the head

Subarachnoid bleed - Bleeding between two layers of the coating of the brain. The rupture of an aneurysm often brings this on, which is a weak area on the blood vessel that forms into a balloon.

Arthritis—inflammation in blood vessels inside and outside of the head

High blood pressure—most of the time, a mild to moderate amount of high blood pressure does not cause headaches. However, if blood pressure is extremely high, in the range of 180–240 systolic and 100–130 diastolic, headaches can occur.

Arteriovenous malformation—this is a deficit present since birth, in which rather enlarged arteries and veins are joined together. Headaches can occur with or without rupture of these blood vessels, but if they rupture, it is usually a more serious condition.[2]

Migraine Disease

It is by and large a hereditary disease that starts at adolescence in 35 percent of patients. By the age of twenty-five years, 60 to 70 percent of patients with migraine disease start having migraines. Some start getting the headaches after the age of twenty-five. If someone gets the onset of headaches after fifty years of age, the condition should be viewed with suspicion and investigated well. One exception is that cluster headaches can occur after the age of fifty and are not that uncommon. Clinically, the headaches are usually on one side and associated with nausea, vomiting, sensitivity to light and sound, dizziness, low blood pressure, and fainting spells. Some patients get an

---

2 Stephen Silberstein, Richard Lipton, and Peter Goads by *Headache in Clinical Practice.*

aura before the headache in the form of loss of vision, shimmering vision, numbness, weakness, trouble speaking, and so forth. At first, the attacks are only one to two times a month but gradually increase to three to four times a week. There are many precipitating factors that tend to bring on headaches, which include missing a meal, alcohol, too much caffeine, ripe cheeses, pork, hot dogs, monosodium glutamate (MSG; present in Asian food), chocolate in large amounts, caviar, dry fish, spoiled meat, broad beans, and so forth; too much or too little sleep; exercise or sexual activity; and stress of a physical or psychological nature.

Even if the majority of the criteria are present and neurological examination is negative, one can still not be 100 percent certain about a diagnosis of migraines. Over the years, I saw roughly three patients a year in which a diagnosis of something other than migraines was discovered because I was in the habit of obtaining a CAT scan or MRI scan of the brain. Any patient who is being seen for the first time for headaches should ask for a scan.

Diseases Associated with Migraines
Epilepsy
Vertigo (dizziness)
Familial tremors
Asthma
Allergies
Urticaria (hives)
Lichen planus
Depression
Manic-depressive illness
Panic disorders
Anxiety disorders
Irritable bowel syndrome (chronic abdominal pain with alternating episodes of constipation and diarrhea)
Low or high blood pressure
Raynaud's disease (cold hands and feet and pain when touching something cold like an ice cube)

Mitral valve prolapse (the valve between two chambers in the left side of the heart is not placed in its normal position; most of the time, it does not cause any symptoms, but sometimes it causes chest pain, palpitation, heart attacks, and so on) they have migraines sometimes.
Angina and heart attacks
Strokes

Life Cycle of Migraines
It has been formulated that the incidence of migraines increases from the age of three years to forty years. Decrease in migraines begins at the age of fifty or sixty. At the age of seventy, there is a high death rate from migraines, which is roughly two times higher than the normal population. The death rate in women is much lower.

Primary Headache Disorders
Migraine without aura
Migraine with aura
Ophthalmoplegic migraines
Childhood periodic syndromes—intermittent vertigo, intermittent abdominal pain
Complications of migraines

Tension-Type Headaches
Episodic tension-type headaches
Chronic tension-type headaches

Cluster Headaches
Cluster headaches—episodic or chronic
Chronic paroxysmal hemicranias
Idiopathic stabbing headaches
External post-stimulus headaches—ice-cream headaches
Benign cough headaches

Exertional headaches

Headaches associated with exertion and sexual activity

Head trauma

Headaches associated with vascular diseases

Blood clot

Blood in the head with bleeding between two layers of the coverings of the brain

Inflammation of intracranial blood vessels

High blood pressure

CSF—Cerebral spinal fluid pressure (either high or low)

Brain tumors

Raised intracranial pressure

Headaches from substance withdrawal or use

Viral or bacterial infections of the brain

Hypoxia (decreased oxygen) and hypercapnia (increased carbon dioxide in the blood)—low blood sugar, dialysis, and other metabolic factors

Headache or pain associated with disease of the skull, neck, eyes, ears, nose, sinuses, mouth, and teeth

Facial and temporomandibular joint disease—temporomandibular joint disease is like arthritis where the mandible and the temporal bone meet and the pain is caused on one side of the face.

Trigeminal neuralgia—pain of an electric shock quality lasting for a few seconds and occurring up to one hundred times a day

Glossopharyngeal neuralgia—pain in the throat and ears

Occipital neuralgia—pain in the back part of the head

CHAPTER 5

Migraines (General Management)

T he phrase "management of migraine headaches" is much more appropriate than "treatment of headaches." The most important part of treatment is the use of medications. This includes the use of preventive medicines and medicines to get rid of the headache.

There are many other avenues, as listed below:

Change in lifestyle
Curtailing some foods
Stress management in appropriate cases
Psychological evaluation and treatment if necessary
Biofeedback
Acupuncture
Physical therapy
Injections of botulism toxin around the skull
Injections of steroids and local anesthetic between the fifth and sixth vertebrae
New sleep routine if necessary
Avoiding triggers such as excessive heat, exposure to sun, and high altitude

Management of anxiety and depression
Avoiding vigorous exercise

This is a complete list. Only one or a few may be applicable to a given patient.

Change in Lifestyle and Sleep Pattern

If a person has a habit of sleeping too late and getting up too late, it may be a triggering mechanism for migraines. Sleeping at the same time of night and getting up at the same time will avoid headaches. It is not always a good idea to take a nap in the middle of the day because very often it causes headaches. Many people who sleep late on Saturdays and wake up late on Sundays very often wake up with headaches. If they sleep at the same time as weekdays and get up at the same time, they would probably avoid headaches. The alternative treatment is to wake up the same time as weekdays, have a light breakfast, and go back to sleep; most of the time, this will keep the headache at bay. Avoid excessive heat and long exposure to the sun.

Foods to be avoided

A detailed list of food articles is shown on the following pages. I prepared this list for my patients, and it is still up to date. Most of the work needs to be done by the patient. One way is to write down the name of the food that brings on the headache. The other way is to avoid one food at a time and deduce the culprit.

Foods that cause headaches include the following:

Chocolate—dark chocolate is much worse than milk or white chocolate. One should not indulge in more than one or two small pieces.

Cheeses—Avoid cheddar, Swiss, Gouda, Brie, bleu, Roquefort, Stilton, mozzarella, Parmesan, Romano, Boursault, Emmentaler, Camembert, and Gruyère. Cottage cheese and ricotta in moderate amounts are safe.

Other Dairy Products—Buttermilk, yogurt, sour cream, and chocolate milk in large quantities should be avoided.

Alcohol (in all forms)—one can occasionally try one glass of white wine or a drink of vodka, rum, gin, or tequila, well diluted and drunk slowly. If it still causes headaches, you should stop drinking it entirely.

Caffeine—coffee, tea, cocoa, and cola drinks. One or two cups of coffee, tea, cocoa, or two small bottles of cola drinks. Sometimes, these can help headaches. However, if they cause headaches, they should be eliminated. It is not a good idea to stop caffeine abruptly because that can cause severe headaches. I usually advise my patients to stop sip by sip. That is, however, an extreme example.

Meat, fish, and poultry—fresh meat and fish are safe. Pork, however, can cause headaches, and it is much more important in children. Children with a history of migraines should give up pork altogether.

Meat products to be avoided are hot dogs or frankfurters (contain good doses of nitrites and should be avoided), fermented sausages, cured and processed meat, baked ham, pickled herring, caviar, liver (especially chicken liver), bologna, salami, pepperoni, aged ham, salted dried fish, and meat prepared with soy sauce or yeast extract.

Vegetables— Fava beans or broad beans, snow peas, lima beans, lentils, navy beans, pinto beans, garbanzo beans, olives, pickles, onions, and sauerkraut should be avoided.

Fruits and nuts—oranges, grapefruits, tangerines, pineapples, lemons, limes, bananas (only half of a partly green banana is safe), raisins, papayas, passion fruit, avocados, red plums, peanuts and peanut butter, figs, sunflower seeds, sesame seeds, and pumpkin seeds should be avoided.

Bread and cereals—freshly baked yeast bread, doughnuts, sourdough bread, cereals with chocolate and nuts, and pizza are not good to eat.

Soups—bouillon cubes and soup base should be avoided.

Condiments—excessive amount of red pepper should be avoided. Vinegar and foods containing vinegar should be avoided in excess.

Food coloring—some food colorings can cause headaches.

MSG— This is a very important item to avoid. In addition, the following names are used for MSG: hydrolyzed protein, natural flavor and seasoning, and Kombu extract. It's not only Chinese food that involves sauces with MSG, but also Thai, Japanese, Vietnamese, Singaporean, Malaysian, Indonesian, and so forth, that are cooked with soy sauce.

Some other foods—dinner entrées (frozen), canned and dried fruits, potato chips, canned meat, international foods, most diet foods and powders, cured and luncheon meats, most sauces in cans and jars, most salad dressings and mayonnaise, and restaurant food, especially soups, sauces, and salad dressings

Other Treatments

Stress management

Almost every patient, when asked, "What is causing your headache?" invariably answers, "Stress." However, only a few patients require stress management. Many of them can accomplish this at home through gentle exercise and yoga. I personally found swimming, cooking, traveling, and reading nonmedical literature quite ethereal and relaxing. Few patients who are particularly bad may need the help of a psychologist or psychiatrist.

Biofeedback

This technique can be used with both migraine and tension-type headaches. The first part is useful for migraine patients. A single thermometer is attached to a finger, and the psychologist provides some instructions. The idea is to relax and try to imagine a pleasant scene that is true and brings some happiness to you. This should increase the temperature by 7° F. What that does is divert blood flow from the brain to the hand, which in turn decreases the headache. Of course, this does not occur in one day; it is in fact a twelve-week program. Not everyone can accomplish this. I, personally, have difficulty increasing even by 1° F. The second part of the test is to hook the patient to the electromyographic

(EMG) machine. Initially, there is a loss of muscle activity, and one can listen to that. The patient is taught how to relax. Ideally, EMG activity should dwindle quite a bit. If that can be achieved, tension headaches would improve. I also failed this part of the test.

There are two situations where this treatment is most useful: early childhood to late teenagers fare the best because their minds have not been corrupted yet; and pregnant women who cannot take any medication.

Acupuncture
I was treated once with no good results. The procedure involves a long wire being inserted in the head to the arms, first on one side and then the other side. It is not as painful as it sounds. Most patients do respond but only for a couple of months. It has to be repeated at intervals of four to six months. One other drawback, besides life-long treatment, is that medical insurance usually does not pay for this treatment.

Physical therapy
This has many components. Many patients with both migraine and tension-type headaches have spasms in the neck muscles and around the scalp, especially around the front and the sides. Ultrasound, passive and active range of motions, and sometimes tranquilizers do help them with the headaches to some degree. This usually requires about three months of being treated three times a week. If necessary, it can be repeated in a year or so.

Botulism toxin
The toxin is capable of producing temporary paralysis of the muscles. It is given in minute doses around the head. The effect can last two to four months, and then it can be repeated. Because of the relaxation brought by the toxin, the headache tends to improve. It is like physical therapy in some ways.

There are four different preparations:
Botox is onabotulinum toxin A. This has been in use since 1989.

Dysport (abobotulinumtoxina) was first approved in 2009.
    This is prepared from the hollow strain of botulinum.

Xeomin (incobotulinumtoxina) is also prepared from the hollow strain of Clostridium botulinum.
    This was approved in 2010.

Myobloc (rimabotulinumtoxinb) was first approved in 2000.
    This is prepared from botulinum type B.
    This dose varies from one preparation to the next.

Injection of steroids and local anesthetics between the fifth and sixth cervical vertebrae
This was developed by trial and error. This injection gets rid of headaches temporarily for a period of two to four weeks. It can be repeated no more than six times a year. If the injection is given between the first and second vertebrae, this tends to help tension-type headaches.

Management of anxiety and depression
Anxiety and depression are rather common in migraine patients. If the symptoms are mild, they can be treated for a few months with antianxiety medication. Also, if depression is mild, any one of the antidepressants can be used for six months. If the symptoms are severe, patients should be referred to a psychiatrist.

Hypnosis
This can be self-induced or given by a physician; most of the time, it is given by a psychiatrist. Hypnosis is more common during childhood. It works for six months, and then generally headaches quiet down. The technique can be used for a year or so if necessary. This can be combined with medications.

TENS

Transcutaneous electrical neurological stimulation as the name implies, an area of the neck or skull is stimulated continuously with a small electrical current. In some individuals this relieves headaches as long as the stimulus is used. As we have seen with every protocol or procedure, it does fail after a while. After some reasonable interval, it can be reused. The ultimate control is in the hands of the patients, and they can manipulate it when necessary.

Miscilanius Medications

Homeopathic

There are several other chemicals that can be used. The only medicine that is used in homeopathic medicine is Chionanthus virginica. I had the opportunity to take this. It worked like magic for six months, and then it quit working altogether.

Riboflavin

In large doses of 400 mg a day can be effective in some patients. This is vitamin B2 and has no side effects. It is not known exactly how it works, but it has been tried at a number of centers.

CoQ10

Starting with 100 mg a day and gradually increasing to 300mg a day has been shown to be effective in some patients. Some patients feel light-headed and develop loss of coordination, so the dose may have to be reduced to only 100–200mg a day.

Butterbur

There is a poisonous root called butterbur root, which is processed so the poisonous part is taken away. It is presented in the form of capsules of 75mg each. Patients need to be started with just one capsule a day and then increased to 75mg two times a day. It takes about three months to work, but it is supposed to be effective in about 70 percent of patients.

I personally could not take CoQ10, but I am taking riboflavin (vitamin B2) 400mg a day and butterbur 150mg a day with lessening in the severity of my headaches.

Treatment of Migraines

The non-medicinal methods have been outlined previously. Of course, these methods can be used with medicines. Drug treatment is, however, the mainstay of treatment in migraine headaches.

Before I embark on the drug treatments, a few other points need to be made.

Medications Causing Headaches

There are a variety of drugs that cause headaches as side effects. These should be avoided; one can always substitute another medicine. Surprisingly, some of these medications are for the prevention or acute treatment of headaches, so one has to weigh the evidence.

Calcium Channel Blockers

These calcium channel blocking drugs are extremely useful in the prevention of migraines and cluster headaches. Fortunately, verapamil is the most commonly used drug in this group and has a fairly low incidence of headaches.

Verapamil	9%
Cardizem	8%
Procardia	9%
Adalet	23%
Nimotop	3%

Nonsteroidal Anti-Inflammatory Drugs

Arthritis Pills
This group is quite satisfactory because of its low incidence of headaches.

Ibuprofen	4%
Naprosyn	6%
Indocin	12%
Tolectin	6%
Dolobid	6%
Voltaren	6%
Meclomen	6%
Ovudis	6%
Celebrax	5%
Vioxx	5%

Cardiac Vasodilators—Drugs to Open Arteries of the Heart

Fortunately, we do not use much of this group.

Isordil	25%
Nitroglycerin	50%
Nitrolingual spray	50%
Sorbitrate	25%

High Blood Pressure Medication
This group is pretty satisfactory, but neurologists do not use many of these medications. I would first try beta-blockers or calcium channel blockers, which help headaches the most.

Lopressor	10%
Minipress	8%
Minizide	8%

Moduretic	6%
Tenex	3%
Vasorectic	5%
Viotension	5%
Vesterectese	5%
Zestril	5%

Antiviral Medications

Mexidal	7%
Ritrovil	30%
Zovirax	4%

Hormones

Lupron injections	6%
Cholesterol-lowering agents	10%
Meclovil	12%
Multiple sclerosis therapy	12%

Psychotropic Medications

Clozaril	6%
Prozac	20%
Xanax	13%
Halcion	10%
Ludiomil	5%

Antispasticity

Lioresal	6%
Hytran	11%

Analgesic Injections

Nubain   2.5%
Stadol   2.5%

Anti-Parkinson's Medications

Permax   5%
Parlodel   15%

Antiallergy Tablets

Seldane   16%

CHAPTER 6

Food in Different Countries and Migraines

There are many parts of the world that have much less incidence of migraines. The causes are multifactorial. It is well established that the incidence of migraines in the United States and many Western European countries is much higher. Many foods in different countries can precipitate migraines.

Spain

Aguardiente—made from musk Madeira and flavored with anise
Bisque—shellfish puree with white wine, cognac, and fresh cream, Both
of these can cause severe headaches.

China

The incidence of migraines is only 0.63 percent. The only pertinent thing that causes headaches in the Chinese is monosodium glutamate (MSG) used in many of their food preparations.

Greece

Brewer's yeast used in baked goods
Cider—fermentation of apple juice in the form of cider
Ouzo—liquor from anise
All of these are capable of causing severe headaches.

Germany

Bock—dark, strong beer
Diplomat pudding—rum and kirsch pudding
Diplomat cream and dried fruits
These three are examples of what cause headaches in some Germans foods.

France

The incidence of migraines in France is only 5 percent.
>   Anchovies
>   April food—fat chocolate and marzipan
>   Atriaux—sausage, pork liver, veal, onions, and herbs
>   Brandy—spirits distilled from wine such as cognac, which is actually made from grapes
>   Figs and red wine

Switzerland

The incidence of migraines in Switzerland is 14 percent.
>   Cheese
>   Aquavit—flavored liquor distilled from grain
>   Buttermilk
>   Fondue (especially cheese and chocolate)

Poland

Baba—cake made from dough containing raisins, rum, and kirsch syrup

Africa

Agraz—a combination of almonds, verjuice, sugar, and kirsch

Boukha—a Tunisian spirit made from figs and drunk as a digestive aid, served in North Africa with kola nut. Kola nuts are rich in caffeine and are used for making cola drinks. They are chewed for their stimulant effect

India

The incidence of migraines in India is 2 percent. Differences in geography, cultures, genetics, and ethnicities have resulted in differences in the food. The special foods of India are tamarind, rich and heavy foods, pork consumed by Hindus, and large amounts of yogurt and red chilies. There are also differences in lifestyle, such as afternoon naps. Siestas lead to less stress, which is a major contributor to headaches.

CHAPTER 7

Prevention and Treatment of Migraines

For a period of about thirty years (1960s–1980s), the only medicine used for acute attacks was Fiorinal (aspirin, caffeine, and butalbital), a kind of rapid-acting barbiturate. Later, another medicine was created, Fioricet (acetaminophen, caffeine, and butalbital). These remain popular medications. Later, they added one quarter of a grain of codeine so that it could be used for more severe headaches. It is worth emphasizing that not every patient requires similar medications. It should be a tailor-made approach. In the same patient, many different medications may be used for different kinds of attacks. For example, for mild to moderate headaches, one can use aspirin, Tylenol, or nonsteroidal anti-inflammatory drugs (NSAIDs). For more severe cases, ergotamine or dihydroergotamine (DHE) are used. It is best to avoid narcotic drugs because of the chronicity of the problem, and many patients become used to these. Also, an increasing amount of medication is necessary if the headaches are chronic. They do, however, work for neck, chest, and abdominal pain. Percocet is a combination of oxymorphone; this is usually a combination of oxycodone 7.5mg and acetaminophen (Tylenol) 325mg. Unfortunately, once this pain pill is taken, it becomes ineffective in subsequent attacks. Percodan is a much stronger pill than Percocet, which has oxycodone 4.5mg, hydrocodone 5–10mg, and aspirin 325mg. Other narcotics and somewhat detailed accounts will be discussed at a more appropriate juncture.

By and large, preventive treatment is very effective in the prevention of migraine headaches. The number of drugs has mushroomed and cannot be counted on the fingers of both hands. I will discuss them later in great detail, but here I will just mention the major ones. NSAIDs are used for prevention as well as acute treatment of migraines in some patients. Other medications such as beta-blockers, calcium channel blockers, antidepressants (amitriptyline, Vivactil, Nardil, Effexor, etc.), and antiepileptic drugs (zonisamide, Neurontin, Topamax, etc.) are also used for prevention.

Nonsteroidal Anti-Inflammatory Drugs

This class of drugs is used mainly for the treatment of osteoarthritis and rheumatoid arthritis. By trial and error, it was found that these NSAIDs can be used for acute treatment as well as preventive-type treatment of migraines, tension-type headaches, cluster headaches, menstrual headaches, headaches from exertion, cough headaches, and headaches related to sexual activity.

Generic Name	Average Dose	Arthritis Medications Very Useful in Different Kinds of Headache Patients
Acetaminophen (Tylenol)	1,400	Liver toxicity, genetics.
Aspirin	975	Toxicity is mostly irritation of the stomach and hyperacidity.
Diflunisal	1,000 twice a day	Gastrointestinal toxicity, genetics.
Ibuprofen	1,200	Good for prevention as well as treatment of headaches.
Indocin (indomethacin)	20–150 a day	This can also be given by rectal suppository. This medicine has been used for cluster headaches, paroxysmal hemicranial pain, stabbing headaches, and so forth.
Flurbiprofen	100	Treatment of acute headaches.
Ketoprofen	150	Can be used through intramuscular injection as well as acute treatment of headaches by mouth.
Naproxen	500	Good medication for prevention and acute attacks.
Sulindac	300	Low kidney toxicity.
Suprofen	600	Low toxicity.
Tolmetin	600	Liver toxicity is still quite low.
Piroxicam	20	Treatment of acute headaches.
Mefenamic acid	400 a day	Can cause bone marrow toxicity.

Tylenol—initial dose is two 325mg tablets. It is quite safe. If the dose is exceeded and the person drinks a lot of alcohol, it can cause liver failure. Tylenol is especially useful in children and often used in a small dose during pregnancy. Some adults do respond to Tylenol, three to four tablets of 325mg each with caffeine. In patients with a rather systemic illness of some severity, Tylenol will probably be a safe medication.

Aspirin—initial dose is 1,400mg. It has a higher incidence of hyperacidity and peptic ulcer disease.

Ibuprofen (Motrin)—a dosage of two tablets of 200mg is fairly safe. Some patients can have small bleeding blisters and gastrointestinal symptoms associated with ibuprofen. Ibuprofen is useful in children. It also works as a short-term prophylactic agent. If children decide to play tennis in warm weather, they can take 200–400mg of ibuprofen, thirty minutes before a game. For some women, ibuprofen can help menstrual migraines.

Naproxen—this is available in the form of tablets and suspension. Of all the NSAIDs, this is the most useful for menstrual headaches. A dose of 500mg twice a day is usually enough. If this could be started a day or two before the cycle and continued for a day or two after the cycle, many times the menstrual headaches can be avoided. Its efficacy is around 70 percent.

Indomethacin (Indocin)—this is available in the form of tablets and suppositories. Its uses include cluster headaches, paroxysmal hemi-cranias, intermittent stabbing pain, cough headaches, headaches as-sociated with sexual activity, and headaches from physical exertion. A large dose of NSAIDs can be rather hard on the stomach for some pa-tients, resulting in abdominal pain, vomiting, anemia, and dizziness.

Ketorolac—this is found to be of the same strength as meperidine (Demerol). A dose of 60mg of ketorolac intramuscularly is equal to 75mg of Demerol and one of the antinausea medicines, such as 25mg of Phenergan (promethazine).

Collectively, these medicines are useful in moderate degrees of head-aches. Side effects of this group include nausea, vomiting, abdominal cramps, and diarrhea, small blood spots on the skin and aplastic anemia, and loss of red cells, white cells, and platelets. These side effects can be easily reversed.

Ergot in the Treatment of Migraines

In the middle ages, grains contaminated with ergot (*Claviceps purpurea*) caused epidemics of gangrene, known as holy fire. It has sympathetic ac-tivity because ergot can cause constriction of blood vessels, also known as vasoconstriction. This particular activity with constriction of blood ves-sels is what helps headaches. The drug dihydroergotamine (DHE) was introduced as a treatment modality in 1945. DHE was found to be more potent than ergotamine itself.

Alkaloids have a complex mode of action. They work on 5-hydroxy-tryptamine (5HT), dopamine, and noradrenaline receptors.

Marked vasoconstriction is seen with ergotamine and DHE in carotid arteries. Besides that, it has some action on peripheral cerebral (brain), temporal, and coronary arteries.

Clinical Usefulness of Ergotamine and DHE

Ergotamine is still used in many countries in a dose of 2–3mg given intramuscularly (the intravenous route causes intense nausea and vomiting). One should take one of the anti-nausea medications (Reglan, Compazine, or Thorazine) half an hour beforehand. Cafergot, which consists of 1mg of ergotamine and 100mg of caffeine, can work well in some patients. Of course, it takes longer to act that way. There is a preparation for rectal use, which has 2mg of ergotamine and 100mg of caffeine. Because rectal absorption is better than the oral route, this is more effective.

Ideally, no more than two doses should be used in a week. Taking more than that causes persistent constriction, habit formation, and daily headaches. Patients with auras—especially if the auras last more than thirty minutes—should avoid ergotamine.

Side Effects of Cafergot

Side effects include nausea, vomiting, abdominal pain, acroparesthesia (tingling and numbness in the hands and feet), swollen fingers, leg cramps, diarrhea, tremors, syncope, and symptoms of angina (heart pain).

Chronic Daily Intake of Cafergot

Ergotamine-induced chronic headaches and ergotamine-withdrawal headaches occur in people who take these medications on a regular basis. It also causes blue discoloration of the legs, acroparesthesia, and anorectal ulcers from too much use of suppositories, and ischemic neuropathy (neuropathy from poor circulation).

DHE in Acute Treatment of Headaches

This is given as a 1 mg intramuscular or subcutaneous injection; sometimes, it can also be given as a smaller dose, such as 0.5mg intravenously. These patients should also be given something for nausea beforehand. A nasal spray preparation is now available, which can be effective in some patients.

The most common side effects are nausea, leg pain, angina, and ergot toxicity. It is better to use one of the anti-nausea medications, particularly with the intravenous dose, to be given thirty minutes beforehand. Side effects of the nasal spray include nasal congestion, nausea, and throat discomfort.

Triptans- 5-HT1B/1D Receptor Agonists in the Treatment of Migraines

Triptans are a new class of drugs that are similar in action to 5-hydroxytryptamine. The first one, called sumatriptan, came out in 1991 and was a great advancement in the treatment of migraine therapy. Initially, it came as an injection, and after about six months, it came in the form of tablets. Other drug companies came out with six different triptans over a period of about ten years.

Drug	Comments	Headache Response (%)
Sumatriptan nasal spray 20 mg	Very effective	68
Sumatriptan 100 mg tablet	Has a rather short half-life	65
Sumatriptan subcutaneous 6 mg	Sometimes it causes fleeting, tingling chest pain, and palpitations.	80
Zolmitriptan 2.5 mg	Patients taking monoamine oxidase inhibitors (MAOIs) can take up to 5 mg a day.	62
Rizatriptan 10 mg	It seems to work faster than most other triptans.	66
Naratriptan 25 mg	Has a long half-life; it is more useful in patients with menstrual migraines.	49
Almotriptan 25 mg	Has longer life.	63
Frovatriptan 40 mg	Has fairly long life.	30
Eletriptan 40 mg	Has longer life.	60

All these triptans work the same way. They can relieve headaches in 40 to 80 percent of migraine patients. Their side effects are similar but not identical. These include tingling in the head, headaches, tingling in the arms and legs, palpitations, and so on. The side effects of zolmitriptan, or Zomig, which was the second triptan introduced in the United States, are weakness, nausea, sleepiness, dizziness, tingling, and numbness in the extremities.

In general, triptans are rather effective drugs for treatment of acute attacks of migraines. The drugs are by and large safe, and side effects of all are rather mild and predictable. There are a few precautions that are necessary to take. These drugs should not be used in patients with uncontrolled hypertension and a history of significant coronary artery disease or use of MAOI drugs, which are usually used for difficult patients with depression. The exception to the rule is Zomig, which can be used up to 5mg a day with Nardil or other MAOIs.

The following are some other considerations about treatment with triptans. They can be used between the ages of eight and fifty. I have, however, treated some children as young as six years old, and even though age fifty is the usual cutoff, patients have taken triptans up to the age of sixty as long as they do not have severe hypertension or coronary artery disease. Naratriptan and frovatriptan are two triptans that have long lives and when given one tablet two times a day can be a good regime for menstrual migraines. The length of treatment depends on the number of days of menstrual migraines.

Only two tablets of triptans can be used within a span of twenty-four hours. If that does not work, some other pain medications, including narcotics, may have to be tried. One tablet of triptan costs fifteen to twenty dollars. If a person gets four headaches a week, and some may require two tablets a day, the total cost may be staggering. Some insurance companies cover these triptan drugs, while others do not.

Combination Triptan → Treximent

This is a combination of sumatriptan 85mg and naproxen 500mg, which is a nonsteroidal anti-inflammatory agent. Treximet came on the market in mid-2008. Treximet is approved to treat migraines with aura and migraines without aura in adults.

It seems to work better than sumatriptan alone. It is also faster, and the side effects are minimal.

Opiates (Pain Medications)

In chronic conditions like migraines, it is best to avoid opiates. Short-term opiates are useful to treat attacks of migraines that are quite severe in nature. There are two inherent properties of these drugs. As one keeps taking the medicine, larger and larger doses are required. Despite taking larger and larger doses, the efficacy or response to the medication becomes less and less. If compared to more conventional types of anti-migraine drugs such as Motrin, aspirin, Tylenol, and triptan, they all seem to work at the same dose even ten years after some have started the medication, and there is very little drug abuse.

Opiates	Comments
Butorphanol 1 mg	Repeat same in one to two hours
Hydrocodone 5 mg and Tylenol 650 mg (Vicodin)	Can be repeated on PRN basis
Meperidine (Demerol) 100 mg oral dose to 50–100 mg intramuscularly	Will help most of the time
Methadone 20 mg	Given several times a day
Morphine 60 mg	Repeated after a while with 30 mg
Oxycodone 15 mg (OxyContin)	This is a rather long-acting drug that can be taken two times a day and can be part of a pain-management program. It was once recorded as having strong addiction potential. Unfortunately, the value of the drug on the street is fifteen to twenty times more than its purchase value, which makes seeking these drugs and criminal behavior much more frequent.

In resistant cases when patients who do not respond to any medication, 1.5mg of Decadron twice a day for three days can break the cycle. For hydrocortisone the usual dose needed is 100mg given intravenously every eight hours for a period of three days, which would usually break the cycle.

The following medications are used for nausea and vomiting:

Many patients with severe migraines get nausea and vomiting. It is a good idea to give something for nausea before some kind of pain medicine is given.

Reglan (metoclopramide) can be given intramuscularly or intravenously and has very few side effects.

Phenergan (promethazine) 25–50mg can be taken by mouth, intramuscularly, intravenously, or rectally. It is quite effective but causes some degree of drowsiness.

Vistaril (hydroxyzine) in a dose of 25–50mg is quite effective. This can be given by mouth, by the intramuscular route, or by the intravenous route.

Thorazine (chlorpromazine) is basically an antipsychotic medication but has good antinausea and antivomiting properties. It is usually given intramuscularly or by mouth.

*Reglan, Thorazine, Stelazine, Phenergan, and Compazine, when given intravenously, can sometimes get rid of the headache without using any pain medications.

Zofran was introduced more than ten years ago for nausea and vomiting in cancer patients. It does work for nausea and vomiting in a dose of 4mg by mouth or intravenously but does not help headaches.

There are many medications that are under trial for treatment of migraines. These include the following:

5-HT1B/1B receptor agonists
Selective 5-HT1B receptor agonists
Selective 5-HT1F receptor agonists
5-HT1F receptor agonists
CGRP receptor antagonists
Neurokinin 1 (NK1) receptor agonists
Spreading depression antagonists
Drugs effective against nitrous oxide

One of the drug categories that were mentioned previously (CGRP receptor antagonists) includes a medicine called telcagepant 150mg to 300mg. Not much is known about this medication yet.

Stimulation of the Scalp (Non Medical Treatment)

Low-current stimulation of the scalp, usually in the frontal area, has been found to be useful in getting rid of headaches in some patients. This is done through a metallic plate. This is similar to transcutaneous electrical nerve stimulation (TENS) used in the spinal cord for low back pain.

Treatment of Prodromes and Aura

Prodromes are symptoms that occur a day or two before headaches. A drug by the name of domperidone 40mg given at the onset of a prodrome can often eliminate the prodrome as well as the headache. For treatment of the aura, 10 percent carbon dioxide plus 90 percent oxygen inhaled for five minutes is temporarily effective. One hundred percent oxygen inhaled for about one hour produced 42 percent relief of headaches. Nifedipine 10 mg given sublingually (under the tongue) can be effective in getting rid of the aura.

Lasix (a water pill) is effective in preventing the aura, as are steroids, Thorazine, and intravenous magnesium. They can not only prevent the aura but also help with the headaches.

Comparison Of Triptans

When it comes to treatment in a given patient with migraines, only certain medications can be used. Sometimes, the first medication works; other times, it is trial and error. The table below provides a perceptive list, and at the end I will make some pertinent comments.

This chart shows a comparison of effectiveness, side effects, and cost. A rating of 1+ is least effective, and 3+ are most effective. Side effects are least with 1+, moderate with 1–2+, and most with 4+. This same scale applies to cost as well.

Triptans	Efficacy	Side Effects	Cost
Sumatriptan tablets	3+	1–2+	4+
Intranasal sumatriptan	3+	1–2+	4+
Subcutaneous injection	4+	2+	5+
Zolmitriptan	3+	1–2+	4+
Naratriptan tablet	2+	1+	4+
Rizatriptan	3+	1–2+	4+
Rizatriptan wafer	3+	1–2+	4+
Almotriptan	3+	1–2+	4+
Eletriptan	3+	2+	4+
Frovatriptan	2+	2+	4+
Ergot Alkaloids			
Ergotamine tablet	1–2+	2+	2+
Suppository	3+	3+	2+
Injections	3+	4+	2+
Dihydroergotamine injection	3+	2+	2+
Intranasal	2+	2+	2+

Nonsteroidal Anti-Inflammatory Agents

A detailed description was provided earlier in this chapter. However, just to recap, naproxen is most useful in migraines related to the menstrual cycle but is also a good idea for migraines. Motrin (ibuprofen) is a good medication for children if Tylenol fails. It can be used before participating in competitive sports. An injection of ketoprofen is almost as strong as 50–75mg of Demerol. Indomethacin can be used in some children with headaches but can also be used in cluster headaches, intermittent stabbing headaches, cough headaches, and headaches associated with sexual activity and exercise.

Narcotics

These are best avoided because of the problem of addiction. They are usually effective if taken once in a while.

Prophylactic Management or Prevention of Migraines

The following circumstances demand the use of prophylactic treatment:

Patient has more than two or three attacks per month.
Patient has devastating attacks that impair normal activity.
Patient is emotionally disabled.
Acute treatment does not work or causes serious side effects.
Sometimes, the person's vocation may be such that taking one day out of a month would be too much for him or her.

These prophylactic medications are not to be used by pregnant women. Prophylactic treatment is given for six to twelve months. When the patient is stable, treatment can be stopped. If the headaches come back, the prophylactic treatment can be continued. If the prophylactic quits working after six months to two years, it is time to change the drug. The number of prophylactic medications that are used is so many that one has to choose them judiciously. Ideally, one should start with a single medication. However, if it is not working, one can go with two medications.

Preventive Medications

Phenelzine (Nardil)

Phenelzine (Nardil) is a very old antidepressant. It raises the level of serotonin, dopamine, epinephrine, and norepinephrine. It is a very effective medicine for prophylaxis for migraines. Its dose is 15mg three times a day, sometimes four times a day. It produces anxiety in some patients and manic reactions in others. The food precautions are more or less like the migraine food precautions.

When I took this medicine, on the fifth day my headaches were gone. I had to be careful of such foods as alcohol, too much coffee or cocoa, raspberries, and cough and cold medications. If the medicine works, it is likely to work for a long time.

Bellergal Spacetabs

This is a combination of ergotamine, caffeine, belladonna, and barbiturates. The initial dose is one tablet two times a day, and it can be increased to two tablets two times a day. Its side effects include dry mouth, drowsiness, and pale hands. It takes several weeks before the medication starts to work. Unfortunately, it works in only 40 to 50 percent of patients. It also quits working in six months to a year.

Beta-Blockers

The true concept of prophylaxis started with the introduction of beta-blockers. There was a patient in a Miami hospital that had serious coronary artery disease. Once beta-blockers were introduced around 1970, he was given the first dose of Inderal. He had a lifelong history of migraine headaches. Along with the improvement of his heart disease, his migraines also improved. This drug was tried in many centers with equally good results.

Beta-blockers reduce the vasodilation phase of the blood vessels. They also work by inhibiting, or stopping, serotonin receptors.

The side effects of these drugs include drowsiness, fatigue, sleep disorders, nightmares, depression, memory disturbance, and hallucinations. That said, these side effects are rather uncommon.

Name	Dose (mg)	Efficacy (%)
Blocadren (timolol)	10–40	72
Corgard (nadolol)	40–240	70
Inderal (propranolol)	40–400	68
Lopressor (metoprolol)	50–300	65
Tenormin (atenolol)	50–200	62

These drugs may become important in the prevention of migraine headaches. One of the drawbacks is that the medicines quit working in six months to two years. It is also worth mentioning that not all beta-blockers are alike. If one does not work, it is likely that the others would.

One can sometimes even use a combination of two of them. Once the medication quits working, it can be restarted after six months or so.

There are some conditions where beta-blockers should not be used. Asthma is the most important medical condition where beta-blockers should not be used at all, as well as depression, congestive heart failure, and Raynaud's syndrome (where hands and, rarely, feet become blue and spotty, and touching a cold surface produces intense pain).

Antiserotonin Drugs in Prophylaxis

Pizotifen is a potent $5\text{-}HT_2$-receptor antagonist. It also has antiallergic and antidepressant properties. It improves migraines in the neighborhood of 58 percent. The initial dose is 0.5mg three times a day to be increased to 1.5mg three times a day. This is a dopamine reuptake antagonist. Side effects include nausea, gastrointestinal complications, dizziness, and sometimes Parkinson's-type symptoms. This medicine is not available in the United States.

Periactin (cyproheptadine) has antiallergic and 5-H2 antagonist properties. It is a useful prophylactic agent for migraines in children. After the age of eight to ten, it is usually not very effective. The initial dose is 4mg two times a day to be increased to 8mg three times a day if necessary. The success report is around 50 percent. Side effects include drowsiness, dizziness, dry mouth, and weight gain.

Calcium Channel Blockers (Calcium Antagonists)

Five to six years after beta-blockers were introduced, calcium channel blockers were introduced. Their primary function was treatment of high blood pressure and certain heart conditions. However, they are also very important for prophylaxis of migraines and some other kinds of headaches. These drugs work on smooth muscles of blood vessels and regulate their tone. They also block calcium from getting into blood vessels.

Name	Dose (mg)
Diltiazem	90–270
Flunarizine	Not available in the United States
Nicardipine	90–120
Nifedipine	30–90
Nimodipine	60–120
Verapamil	240–480

Verapamil

It is effective in 70 percent of patients with migraine prophylaxis including migraines with aura. One should wait for eight weeks before deciding if the drug is effective. Side effects occur in about 30 percent of patients. These include constipation, numbness in the arms and legs, abdominal distress, and enlarged breasts in men.

Diltiazem

This drug has not been tried much. Side effects include gastrointestinal distress, rash, edema, and headaches.

Nifedipine

There is about 70 percent improvement with migraines as well as migraines with aura. Side effects include low blood pressure, redness of the face and body, gastrointestinal distress, and headaches.

Nimodipine

When introduced, it was used for management of cerebral bleeding in the head. It reduced the ability to bleed by causing constriction (narrowing) of blood vessels. Subsequently, it was tried in the prevention of migraine headaches and did work in about 60 percent of patients. The only side effect is low blood pressure. It is also extremely expensive.

Antidepressants

Antidepressants are very important drugs for prophylactic treatment of migraines. About 30 percent of patients with migraines have depression. Sleep disturbance is very common in as much as 50 percent of patients. On top of that, many antidepressants help with migraine and tension-type headaches.

Antidepressants can be divided into three categories. This division is chronological (time based).

Nardil

For the last fifty years, Nardil has been used in some special cases of depression where other medications did not work. It works by increasing dopamine, 5-hydroxytryptamine (5HT), epinephrine, and norepinephrine. This is also an excellent migraine prophylactic medication. The dose and side effects have been discussed previously. This medicine hampers sleep, and sometimes that is a problem.

Tricyclic Antidepressants

These drugs are thirty to forty years old and very useful in terms of treatment of migraines.

Generic Name	Brand Name	Dosage (mg)
Amitriptyline	Elavil	25–50
Clomipramine	Anafranil	100–250
Desipramine	Norpramin	150–300
Doxepin	Adapin	180–300
Imipramine	Tofranil	150–300
Maprotiline	Ludiomil	150–200
Nortriptyline	Pamelor	50–150
Protriptyline	Vivactil	15–60
Trazodone	Desyrel	50–600
Trimipramine	Surmontil	150–300

The star in this group is amitriptyline. First of all, amitriptyline reduces headaches to the greatest degree, and it makes patients sleep much better. The dose has to be escalated slowly. Imipramine is meant for children. Pamelor is another drug for patients who cannot tolerate amitriptyline. It is also useful in the elderly. Vivactil is usually good for adolescents. Desyrel is a good, solid medication but not very effective in migraines.

The side effects of these drugs include drowsiness, tremors, sweating, blurred vision, constipation, low blood pressure, confusion, weight gain, and sexual dysfunction. If these side effects are too bothersome, changes in dose or medication is advised.

Selective Serotonin and Tricyclic Reuptake Inhibitors
These are the latest in the group of antidepressants introduced between fifteen to twenty years ago. Because serotonin is at the base of migraine headaches, it was anticipated that selective serotonin and tricyclic reuptake inhibitors would be extremely fertile in the prevention of migraines. As trials took place at a number of medical centers and universities, their role was found to be very poor. They did little in

preventing migraines. However, they did a little better in prevention of tension-type headaches. They were also fairly good antidepressant medications.

Generic Name	Brand Name	Dosage (mg)
Bupropion	Wellbutrin	200-300
Citalopram	Celexa	10–40
Escitalopram	Lexapro	10–20
Fluoxetine	Prozac	20–80
Mirtazapine	Remeron	15–60
Paroxetine	Paxil	10–40
Sertraline	Zoloft	50–200
Venlafaxine	Effexor	75–300

The side effects are similar in all of these drugs. Prozac and Zoloft make it difficult for a person to sleep. These two drugs also cause weight loss. Remeron, Effexor, and Wellbutrin can cause sleeplessness. They can cause tiredness, rapid heart rate, sweating, blurred vision, low blood pressure, confusion, tremors, and sexual dysfunction.

Of this group, Effexor and Remeron are the most useful in terms of prophylaxis of migraines.

Anticonvulsants (Antiepileptic Drugs)

Antiepileptic drugs have been used for the last seventy years or so. The first four were not very effective. About twenty years ago, a drug came on the market by the name of valproate, which was drastically better than the others. In the last ten years or so, there have been some excellent new drugs with good efficacy for prophylaxis of migraines. About 15 percent of patients with migraines have epilepsy, and by use of this group of drugs, one can take care of both. The side effects of these new antiepileptic drugs are rather mild and often temporary. If we take the three major groups of drugs, namely beta-blockers, calcium channel blockers, and antiepileptic medications and were to run a competitive race, there would be no consistent first or third. If we trace the history of the last fifty to sixty years, the only drug with some promise was monoamine oxidase inhibitors (MAOIs), namely Nardil, with terrible side effects, awful restrictions of food, and so forth.

Phenobarbital and bromide mixture was the first antiepileptic medication. It was not a very strong drug, but it did work in some patients to some degree. Phenobarbital was introduced before World War II. It is a good antiepileptic medication, but its use has fallen by the wayside in the last twenty years or so. In the past, before the newer antiepileptic medications, it was used for fifty years. It was used in children for prophylaxis of migraines with marginal effectiveness. Twenty percent of children developed hyperactivity and irritability. The efficacy for migraine prophylaxis was only about 20 percent.

Primidone (**Mysoline**) is a reasonable drug for the treatment of epilepsy. It is often used in conjunction with phenobarbital and Dilantin. It is of no use in management of migraines.

Carbamazepine (**Tegretol**) was approved for seizures in 1974. The drug was found to be quite versatile and was the most potent antiepileptic drug at that time. It also was used for neuralgic pains such as trigeminal neuralgia. It was found to be useful in many depressive diseases, but as an anti-migraine agent, it was not very effective.

The side effects of carbamazepine (Tegretol) include nausea, vomiting, drowsiness, dizziness, headache, agitation, anxiety, restlessness, skin rash, and a decreased count of all blood cells.

Tegretol was not found to be of much use in the prevention of migraines.

Valproate (**valproic acid, Depakote**) was approved for treatment of epilepsy in 1978. It was found to be a wonderful drug for most kinds of seizures. It could also be used in children without much problem. This turned out to be the first antiepileptic drug that was extremely effective for migraine prophylaxis. It produced its effects by gamma-aminobutyric acid levels.

I presented a paper on the role of Depakote and the prophylaxis of migraine patients. Sixty-nine percent of patients revealed marked improvement. This was in 1993. Later on, I presented another paper in which there was a 71 percent improvement out of 715 patients.

Depakote is useful in many kinds of epilepsies. The adverse effects are nausea, vomiting, abdominal pain, diarrhea, liver abnormalities, tremors, sleepiness, loss of balance, and high blood ammonia.

Benzodiazepines

These are sedatives and antianxiety medications. In addition, they have anti-seizure properties of varying degrees. The drugs include the following:

Klonopin (clonazepam)
Tranxene (clorazepate)
Valium (diazepam)
Ativan (lorazepam)

Side effects include drowsiness, lethargy, loss of balance, decreased muscle tone, slurred speech, and dizziness. The only usefulness of these drugs in migraines is short-term treatment of anxiety and also short-term treatment for sleeplessness. These are of no use in long-term management of migraines.

Gabapentin (**Neurontin**) was approved by the US Food and Drug Administration (FDA) in 1993. The mechanism of action is not known. It is only moderately effective as far as anticonvulsant properties are concerned. It works to a moderate degree for prevention of migraines; it is also useful in treatment in painful neuralgias and painful neuropathy (painful condition of the legs with tingling, numbness, and burning from diabetes, cancer, or anemia). Side effects include dizziness, sleepiness, and tiredness, which usually go away within three to four weeks.

Lamotrigine (**Lamictal**) was released in the United States in 1994. It is a superb anticonvulsant and works against almost all kinds of seizures. It is not too useful for prophylaxis of migraines, though. The toxic side effects include dizziness, double vision, nausea, and skin rash.

Levetiracetam's (**Keppra's**) mechanism of action is not known. It is a superb drug for prophylaxis of migraines. Its success rate is over 70 percent. Side effects, including drowsiness and dizziness, are quite low.

Tiagabine (**Gabitril**) is an antiepileptic that works on different kinds of seizures. It was introduced in the United States in 1998. It has quite good antimigraine coverage of about 65 percent. The side effects include tremors, sleepiness, and dizziness.

Topiramate (**Topamax**) was approved by the FDA in 1996. It is an excellent antiepileptic. It is also an excellent prophylactic agent against migraines. I have presented a paper regarding 492 patients with an improvement rate of 72 percent.

Zonisamide (**Zonegran**) was approved by the FDA in 2000. This drug is extremely effective in different kinds of seizures. It can also be used in migraine prophylaxis with an improvement rate of 60 to 70 percent. Side effects include sleepiness, loss of appetite, loss of balance, drowsiness, and kidney stones.

Anti-epileptics in Prevention of Migraines

Drug	Improvement in Migraines (%)	Dosage (mg)
Phenobarbital	Children: 20 Adults: 7	Children: 15 bid Adults: 30 bid
Primidone (Mysoline)	5	125–375mg
Carbamazepine (Tegretol)	8	200mg TID
Oxcarbazepine	30	500–1,500mg
Valproate acid (Depakote)	72	500–1,000mg
Gabapentin	49	1,000–2,000mg
Lamotrigine	42	2.5 mg TID
Levetiracetam	74	1,000–2,000mg
Tiagabine	54	500–750mg
Topiramate (Topamax)	69	30–50mg
Zonisamide	63	400–600mg

Miscellaneous Drugs in Prevention of Migraines

MAOI (**Nardil**) has been described previously.

Methysergide (Sansert) was withdrawn from the market in 2004.

Mianserin is a potent 5-H2-receptor antagonist. It does have the potential to be a migraine prophylactic medication. Its efficacy is in the neighborhood of 40 percent.

Cyproheptadine (Periactin) is an antiallergy and anti-5-H2 antagonist. This is especially useful in children for the prophylaxis of migraines. It quits working after the age of eight to ten years. The dose is 2mg three times a day and then gradually increases to 4mg three times a day. Side effects include drowsiness, dizziness, dry mouth, increased appetite, and weight gain.

Clonidine is an antihypertensive medication that works in the lower brain stem. This does work as a prophylactic medication for migraine headaches. The response is in the order of 62 percent in one study and 40 percent in the other study. The initial dose is 0.1mg three times a day and then gradually increases to 0.2mg three times a day. The toxic side effects include low blood pressure, drowsiness, dry mouth, constipation, and occasional disturbance of ejaculation.

Lithium has two important uses. One is the treatment of chronic cluster headaches. Sometimes, when migraine attacks occur for many weeks at a time or they are intermittent—occurring for weeks, going away, and then coming back for a few weeks—lithium can be tried. The average dose is 300mg three times a day. Side effects include kidney problems in the form of poor kidney function, dry mouth, low thyroid condition, and other diseases. It should not be used during the first trimester of pregnancy.

CHAPTER 8

Tension-Type Headaches

Tension-type headaches can be categorized into two different types. One is intermittent, which can last up to forty minutes to ten days. They are nonpulsatile (not throbbing) and not associated with nausea and vomiting but occasionally photophobic (sensitive to light). Some cases are associated with temporomandibular joint dysfunction. Presence of increased tone and muscles around the head are quite common in this group of patients.

Migraines and intermittent tension-type headaches start in adolescence and, oddly, in adulthood. They can also start in childhood. They are more common in women.

Episodic tension-type headaches are much more common than migraine headaches. They are called muscle-contraction headaches due to the thought that there are muscles around the head that have increased tone and because these muscles are what seem to be causing the problem.

There are few medical conditions associated with episodic tension-type headaches. Fibromyalgia is a chronic condition in which pain occurs in the muscles and bones around the head and many parts of the body. It is much more common in women. Patients also have morning stiffness, fatigue, headaches, sleep disturbance, anxiety, and depression. Myofascial pain syndrome is localized and self-limited with trigger points. This means there are several points on the face that are painful when touching or pressing, which is probably related to underlying inflammation.

Biochemistry of Tension Type Headaches

Platelet serotonin, epinephrine (adrenaline), norepinephrine (nor-adrenaline), and dopamine during a headache are decreased.

Genetics of Tension Type Headaches

If one looks into the family history—the parents, siblings, and children—the risk is 3.4 percent more than the general population.

Treatment of Acute Tension-Type Headaches

Simple Analgesics

Aspirin 650mg three to four times a day—most common side effects are hyperacidity (heartburn) and bleeding from the esophagus or stomach.

Acetaminophen (**Tylenol**) 650mg three times a day—there are no significant side effects from this medication except liver problems, which occur only in people who drink excessively.

Nonsteroidal anti-inflammatory drugs—in general, these are more effective than aspirin and acetaminophen. They are also hard on the stomach, resulting in pain, nausea, vomiting, diarrhea, swelling of the liver, and so forth.

A list with doses can be found in pages 58 and 59, "Treatment of Migraines." Lately, there has been much press coverage on so-called COX-2 inhibitors such as Vioxx and Celebrex. These have been implicated in precipitating heart attacks. After a great debate between pharmaceutical companies and the press, the drug companies put the onus on doctors and patients. If there is a history of heart disease, COX-2 inhibitors should not be used.

Combination with Simple Analgesics

A combination of aspirin or acetaminophen with caffeine potentiates or enhances the effects of aspirin and acetaminophen. Taking caffeine for a prolonged period can cause tolerance, habituation, and psychological dependence. Stopping the medicine abruptly can cause withdrawal headaches, dizziness, and irritability. Anacin contains aspirin 400mg and caffeine 32mg. Anacin maximum strength contains aspirin 500mg and caffeine 32mg. Excedrin extra strength contains aspirin 250mg, acetaminophen 250mg, and caffeine 65mg.

The recommended dose for these preparations is two tablets every six hours as needed.

The combination of analgesics with butalbital consists of two very commonly prescribed headache medicines: Fiorinal (aspirin, butalbital, and caffeine) and Fioricet (acetaminophen, butalbital, and caffeine). The recommended dose is also two tablets every six hours as needed. Once again, when taken for a long time, the pills quit working. Also, sudden stoppage of these pills can cause headaches, anxiety, dizziness, and palpitations.

Narcotics in Tension Type Headaches

These should be used as a last resort. It is very easy to get hooked on narcotics. Patients ask for larger and larger doses, despite the fact that the doses do not work for very long periods. Withdrawal is very uncomfortable and can last for a few weeks. Narcotics should be reserved for periods of acute pain, and once that is over, patients should revert back to simple analgesics.

Fiorinal with 15mg of codeine
Fioricet with 30mg of codeine

The dose of both of the above is one capsule every six hours as needed.

Tylenol #3—Tylenol 325mg with codeine 30mg
Tylenol #4—Tylenol 325mg with codeine 60mg
Butorphanol 2mg intramuscular injection is quite effective; butorphanol is also available in a nasal spray of 1 mg by name of Stadol Meperidine (Demerol) oral 50 to 100mg two times a day; injection 50mg two times a day

Hydrocodone contains 7.5mg of hydrocodone plus 500mg of acetaminophen to be taken two to three times a day; these are commonly called Vicodin

Hydrocodone 10mg plus acetaminophen two to three times a day

Ultram and Ultracet (tramadol) can cause nausea and fatigue but are usually well tolerated

Oxycodone (Percocet, Percodan, Tylox, OxyContin) contains 5mg of oxycodeine and aspirin and can be used every three to four hours if necessary

Morphine—the oral dose is 15mg every three to four hours; the injection is given in the form of 10–15mg

Synalgos is a potent narcotic and should be avoided as much as possible. It is a combination of dihydrocodeine 16mg, aspirin 325mg, and caffeine 30mg.

Muscle Relaxants

These are especially useful in patients with a lot of muscle spasms, such as temporomandibular disease, oromandibular disease, fibromyalgia, and trigger points. Muscle relaxants can be used with simple analgesics, pain pills with caffeine, pain pills with butalbital, and various narcotics. They can also be used with nonsteroidal anti-inflammatory agents.

Methocarbamol (**Robaxin**)—works in the brain and is one of the oldest in this class. It begins to work in half an hour, and the action lasts for four to six hours. There is a preparation available with aspirin. The initial dose is 1,000mg followed by 1,000mg every six hours. Side effects are dizziness, headache, blurred vision, and occasional skin rash. Robaxin is available in 500mg and 750mg tablets. Another preparation is Robaxisal, which contains methocarbamol and aspirin 325mg.

Orphenadrine (**Norflex, Norgesic**)-A centrally acting muscle relaxant that reduces muscle spasms and muscle tone. Norflex is available in 100mg long-acting preparations. It is also available in combination with aspirin and caffeine. The dose of Norflex is two times a day. The Norgesic Forte recommended dosage is half to one tablet every eight hours. Side effects include dry mouth, difficulty with urination, rapid heart rate, palpitations, blurred vision, dizziness, constipation, and drowsiness.

Carisoprodol (Soma)- A depressant of the central nervous system, but it does relieve pain and muscle spasms. It has a short duration of action. The dose of Soma is 350mg every six hours. It is also available in combination with aspirin (Soma Compound). It contains 200mg of aspirin and 325mg of carisoprodol. Its dose is one to two tablets every six hours. Another preparation is Soma Compound with codeine. This is 16mg of codeine and Soma Compound. The dose is one to two tablets every six hours as needed.

Chlorzoxazone (**Parafon Forte**)- Available in 250mg and 500mg tablets. Initial dose is 750mg to 2,000 mg in three to four equally divided doses and then 500mg every six hours. Common side effects are dizziness, headaches, nausea, drowsiness, and occasional skin rash.

Metaxalone (**Skelaxin**)-Available in 400mg tablets. The recommended dose is two 400 mg tablets a day. It is usually well tolerated, but it can sometimes cause nausea, dizziness, skin rash, and, very rarely, jaundice.

Special Class of Muscle Relaxants

There is a class of drugs that has properties of tranquilizers, sedatives, and muscle relaxants all in one. In some patients, these drugs might work better than usual muscle relaxants.

Valium (Diazepam) -Available in 2mg and 5mg tablets. The dose can vary from two to three times day to 10 mg three times a day.

Klonopin (Clonazepam) -Available in 0.25mg, 0.5mg, and 1mg tablets. The dose is 0.25 mg three times a day up to 1 mg three times a day.

Xanax (Alprazolam) - Available in doses of 0.25mg, 0.5mg, 1mg, and 2mg tablets. The average dose is 0.25 mg three times a day up to 1 mg three times a day.

Ativan (Lorazepam) -Available in 0.5mg, 1mg, and 2mg doses. The daily dose can be 2–4mg a day into divided doses.

Method of Selecting the Combination of Drugs

It is always a good idea to start with simple painkillers, such as aspirin and acetaminophen, with or without caffeine. If that is not effective, the next thing to try would be a arthritis pills, also known as nonsteroidal anti-inflammatory drugs. One may have to try five or six before finding the one that works. Muscle relaxants and/or tranquilizers can be added to either of the groups. Next in order would be a combination of barbiturates with aspirin or acetaminophen. One should try each medicine for at least one month to see if it is working or not. Finally, narcotics may have to be used if everything else fails.

Other Methods of Treatment

For the last ten to fifteen years, many experts in the field have felt that tension-type headaches are a milder form of migraine headaches. This led to the use of some prophylactic medications that are used for migraines. The most effective is the antidepressant amitriptyline (Elavil). The initial dose is usually 25mg at bedtime. The maximum dose is usually 50–75mg at bedtime. This may reduce the frequency and severity of tension-type headaches in some patients. Nortriptyline (Pamelor) and protriptyline (Vivactil) are reasonably effective. The newer class of antidepressants, such as Prozac, Zoloft, Paxil, Effexor, and so forth, is not as effective as amitriptyline-type drugs, but it does work in some patients.

In this category, there are three other types of headaches that in some manner are akin to chronic tension-type headaches. These include migraines, chronic daily headaches, and headaches from overuse of medication. The distinctions among these headaches are not really clear-cut. The International Headache Society has not defined a clear categorization.

Patients in the chronic-headache group get headaches fifteen days a month. About 5 percent of the general population in the United States, Europe, and Asia get this kind of headache. Patients who take excess amounts of analgesics of any variety are more prone to develop these chronic daily headaches. Medication withdrawal is an important cause of chronic daily headaches.

CHAPTER 9

Chronic Daily Headaches

Primary chronic daily headaches
Chronic migraines
Chronic tension-type headaches
New, daily, persistent headaches

Secondary chronic daily headaches
Posttraumatic headaches
Cervical (neck) spine disorders

Headaches associated with vascular disorders
Arteriovascular malformation
Arthritis (inflammation of blood vessels)
Dissection of artery (tear in the wall of the artery)
Subdural hematoma (formation of blood clot between two layers of coverings of the brain)

Headaches associated with increased pressure in the brain
Infections in the brain

Tumors of the brain

Others such as temporomandibular joint disorders and sinus infections

Chronic Migraines
Some patients who have had difficult migraines all their lives begin to have chronic daily or almost-daily headaches that can pulsate or throb but not too frequently. Only rarely do they have nausea, vomiting, and sensitivity to light and sound. These patients rarely have a history of auras. These chronic migraines usually come on at about sixty years of age but may begin around fifty years of age. Even though the headaches are usually mild, they can be severe at times. Headaches occur at least fifteen times a month. Depression is extremely common in this particular group.

Chronic Tension Headaches
These headaches also occur for about half the month. Pain is dull and more so in the posterior (back) part of the head and neck. Throbbing is almost nonexistent, but some degree of nausea, photophobia, and phonophobia can occur. Pain is mild to moderate and is more a pressure-like sensation.

New Daily Persistent Headaches
These are abrupt in onset and persistent, not lasting for a long period.

Drug-Overuse Headaches
Overuse of analgesics (simple opiate kind of analgesics, preparations, and triptans) can all cause headaches if these medicines are taken on a daily or almost-daily basis. The pain is throbbing in nature and is also associated with nausea, vomiting, photophobia, and phonophobia. Incidence of these varies from 4 to 7 percent.

Rebound Headaches

Caffeine, either in tea or coffee, or caffeine-containing pain pills if suddenly stopped can cause quite severe headaches. It should be tapered and stopped over weeks at a time. Many of the patients take ten to twenty times more barbiturates, two to three times more triptans, and four to five times more narcotics. These drugs eventually cause rebound-type headaches.

There is a significantly higher incidence of depression, anxiety attacks, panic attacks, and manic depressive illnesses in this group. Treating these conditions goes along with rehabilitation of these patients.

Treatment

A gradual decrease of pain medications, triptans, and other preparations are necessary. These medicines cannot be stopped suddenly because the headaches will become much more severe. A period of about six weeks or so is usually a good time to gradually cut off these medicines. In addition to headaches, withdrawal causes anxiety, depression, sleeplessness, perspiration, and sometimes seizures (convulsions). Once this process is completed, patients should try something else that has not been used before. For example, if Midrin, nonsteroidal anti-inflammatory agents, and DHE 45 (dihydroergotamine) have not been used, they can be tried.

Patients also need to be started on a prophylactic (preventive) medication. Any of the prophylactic medications that are used for migraine headaches can be used. These include antidepressants (Elavil, Sinequan, Prozac), beta-blockers (Inderal, Corgard, Blocadren), calcium channel blockers (verapamil, Nimotop), and monoamine oxidase inhibitors (Nardil, which is an antidepressant in a class by itself).

It is also essential to treat existing psychiatric conditions.

Injections of Botulinum Toxin (Botox)

Injections around the skull can be effective in some patients.

CHAPTER 10
Cluster Headaches

Cluster headaches are quite distinct from migraines. Very often, patients do not have a history of these in the family. Sometimes, it is seen in siblings, and very rarely it can occur from parents to children. Compared to migraines, which are much more common in women, cluster headaches are about five to six times more common in men. The disease usually starts in the mid- to late twenties and can continue well into the eighties. These are called cluster headaches because they occur in clusters or bunch. For some reason, these attacks seem to occur more commonly in the fall and spring, and somewhat less frequently in winter. Patients are awakened, usually 90 to 120 minutes after they go to sleep or very early in the morning, such as 4:00 a.m. The pain is so intense that it is thought to be worse than delivering a child. Pain is on one side of the head, and most of the time it remains on the same side. Patients are extremely restless; they cannot lie in bed and usually pace the room. The pain occurs behind the eye, in the temple, and in the frontal area. Patients can develop drooping of the eyelids and smaller-looking pupils on the side of the headache. Some patients become extremely violent and hit the wall or anyone who comes in front of them. Some patients are known to commit suicide during this misery. Fortunately, the pain lasts on average forty-five minutes. Patients can have two to six of these attacks in twenty-four hours. Once the attack starts, it has a tendency to last for about six weeks.

Cluster-headache patients, especially males, have lion like faces, athletic builds, and hazel eyes. Unfortunately, they have low testosterone levels and are rather meek. They can have swelling of the face. Pain from cluster headaches is boring, tearing, or hot burning in the eye, as if the eye is being pushed out, with conjunctival redness and watering of the eye.

Classification

Episodic Cluster Headaches
Chronic Cluster Headaches

Treatment of Episodic Cluster Headaches
They are treated best with a combination of steroids (40–60mg) of prednisone a day and 240–480mg of verapamil a day. If the headaches get milder in seven to ten days, prednisone can be tapered.

Chronic Cluster Headaches

Unfortunately, some patients continue to have cluster headaches for years. Doctors call these chronic cluster headaches. More often, they last for eight to twelve weeks or sometimes nine to twelve months.

Some degree of nausea is observed in 30 percent of patients. Vomiting is distinctly rare. Photophobia can occur in 20 percent of patients.

These are best treated by lithium 600–900mg a day and verapamil 240–480mg a day.

Physical Features

Some patients have deep nasal fissures (a deep furrow between the nose and the face), and the appearance of the skin texture looks like orange peel. They also have a tendency to smoke and drink excessively. High peptic ulceration is quite common.

Psychological Characteristics

A history of head injury is common before the onset of cluster headaches. Neurosis and other psychological anomalies are common. Alcohol, nitroglycerine, and nitric oxide precipitate cluster headaches.

Temporal Arthritis

Temporal arthritis usually starts between fifty-five and sixty years of age. It is caused by an inflammation of blood vessels outside and inside of the head. Most of the pain occurs in the temporal area, hence the name temporal arthritis. The diagnosis can usually be confirmed by a blood test known as sed rate. The sed rate is usually sixty or more. The treatment is usually a high dose of steroids. If that does not stop the process in a matter of four to six weeks, patients may have to be put on one of the anticancer medications that work well with steroids.

Other Cluster-Type Headaches

Trigeminal Autonomic Cephalgia

This consists of a group of headaches associated with head pain in the distribution of the trigeminal nerve.

Hypnic (During Sleep) Headaches

These occur in the elderly, and the pain usually starts 120 minutes after going to sleep. Pain is not as intense as in cluster headaches but can be quite bothersome. Several attacks occur during sleep. Usually, a small dose of lithium 300–600mg a day helps this condition.

Secondary Paroxysmal Hemicrania

The clinical association is that certain diseases responsible are like paroxysmal hemicrania.

Tumor of the sella turcica (where the pituitary gland resides)

Collagen vascular disease

Frontal lobe tumor

Cerebral vascular disease

Cavernous sinus meningioma—a benign tumor that sits behind the
front part of the head and can cause quite severe headaches

Tumor of the parotid—located just below the mandible

Raised intracranial pressure

Paroxysmal Hemicrania Treatment

Indomethacin (**Indocin**) starting with 25mg three times a day and pushing to 75mg three times a day in three to four weeks usually helps the situation. At higher doses, a dose of antacid may have to be added because this is rather hard on the stomach.

Diamox (a water pill) in the dose of 250mg three times a day can be tried.

Imitrex or sumatriptan can be tried in the dose of 100mg, but it has a rather short duration of action.

Arthritis pills (nonsteroidal anti-inflammatory agents) are the next group of drugs to try. Sometimes, verapamil and oxycodone can be tried.

Additional Treatments for Cluster Headaches

If patients are given 100 percent oxygen through a nasal cannula for a period of fifteen to twenty minutes in a sitting position, many patients get relief from their cluster attacks that way.

SUNCT and Trigeminal Neuralgia

SUNCT (short-lasting, unilateral neuralgiform headache attacks with conjunctival injection and tearing) is a very short word for a very long descriptive condition. This is roughly eight times more common in men. The attacks last for five to twenty minutes.

This can be treated with Tegretol, sumatriptan, and indomethacin.

Drug	Dose (mg)
Indomethacin	20
Tegretol	1,200
Sumatriptan (Imitrex)	100
Ergotamine	3
Naproxen	1,200
Ibuprofen or Motrin	1,200
Prednisone	100
Verapamil	Up to 1,500
Lithium	900 a day
Propranolol	150
Amitriptyline	100
Lamotrigine	200
Topamax	200
Lidocaine	Used as a nasal spray

CHAPTER 11

Headaches from Head Trauma

H ead injuries are common in all ages but are most common between adolescence and twenty-five years of age. The symptoms following head injury can occur immediately after injury or after some time. Pain in the neck, shoulders, and head can come on immediately or in twenty-four to forty-eight hours. Pain in the back of the head occurs reasonably early. Some late-onset headaches often take months to manifest.

Sequelae of Mild Head Injuries

Tension headaches
Cluster headaches
Migraine-type headaches
Occipital neuralgia
Low cerebral spinal fluid pressure
Intracranial hypertension
Supracranial neuralgia
Tempomandibular joint dysfunction
Cranial nerve symptoms
Tinnitus and loss of hearing

Diplopia (double vision)

Blurred vision

Light and noise sensitivity

Diminished smell and taste

Other causes including traumatic head or back injury, spinal surgery, and spontaneous cerebrospinal fluid leak

Intracranial hypertension can be associated with swelling of the disc, which is the back part of the eye seen through ophthalmoscope, or it can be not associated with edema or swelling of the optic-nerve head

Secondary hydrocephalus (increased fluid in cavities of the brain)

Neuroblastoma (tumor)

Stroke with hematoma (bleeding)

Meningitis encephalitis

Trauma

Major intracranial venous obstruction

Drugs such as vitamin A, nalidixic acid, antibiotics, and steroids

Renal diseases

Hypoparathyroidism

Uncommon headaches

    Orbital syndromes

    Paracentral syndromes

    Gasserian ganglion syndrome

    Pseudotumor cerebri syndrome (increased pressure in the brain)

CHAPTER 12

Increased Intracranial Pressure

High Spinal Fluid Headaches

High spinal fluid pressure occurs because the spinal fluid in the brain is not absorbed properly. Spinal fluid is produced by specialized structures in the ventricles called choroid plexuses. About 500 cc of spinal fluid is produced in twenty-four hours.

Spinal fluid pressure is measured by doing a spinal tap. Normal pressure is 80mm to 140mm of H_2O. The term *idiopathic intracranial hypertension* is used when there is no obvious cause. It can occur with brain tumors, history of meningitis, stroke and bleeding in the head, and use of too much vitamin A, nalidixic acid, and anabolic steroids.

The diagnosis is made by measuring the spinal fluid pressure. It can range from 250 mm H_2O to 600 mm H_2O.

It occurs in 90 percent of women between the ages of fifteen years to forty years. Most of the patients are overweight. They see their physicians because they have intense headaches. Neurological examination is normal with the exception of swelling of the optic nerve head or papilledema. Some patients lose their vision. Sometimes one of their pupils is larger before their eyesight is disturbed.

Treatment

Weight Loss
It is effective but difficult to do. Some patients opt to have gastric bypass and stapling of the stomach.

Pain Medication-
Pain medication for headaches as and when needed.

Repeated Spinal Tap-
Effective but lasts for only a month or so.

Fluid Restriction-
Some patients do well with fluid restriction, and a low-salt diet helps some patients.

Diuretics-
Diuretics or water pills, Diamox or Acetazolamide, 1–2gram twice a day can be effective for reducing the pressure.

Shunts-
A tube can be put in the subarachnoid space in the lower spinal canal to be drained into the abdominal cavity. It is called a lumboperitoneal shunt.

Alternatively, a plastic tube is put in the lateral ventricle of the brain and drained into the abdomen. Both treatments work, but they have a tendency to get blocked, and surgery has to be repeated.

Optic Nerve Fenestration-

Making a fistula (connecting tube) between the optic nerve head and the subarachnoid space sometimes serves the vision and also helps lower the pressure in some cases.

CHAPTER 13

Headaches in Children and Adolescents

Familial Hemiplegic Migraine

This is characterized by migraines with opposite sides of weakness in the arms and legs. Usually, one of the first-degree relatives has similar attacks. The aura lasts for several hours to three days. In most cases, recovery occurs, but weakness rarely lasts forever. By and large, it is a disease of childhood and adolescence, and attacks disappear after the age of thirty years.

Basilar Artery Migraine

The basilar artery supplies the brain stem and the back part of the brain called the occipital cortex. The English doctor Bickerstaff described this condition.[3]

The auras consist of loss of vision on one side or loss of vision in one quarter of the visual field, dizziness, ringing in the ears, slurred speech, weakness of two or four extremities, numbness of two or four extremities, change in coordination, loss of balance, and so forth.

---

3 Jes Olsen, Peer Tfelt-Hansen, and K. Michael A. Welch, "Basilar Artery Migraines," in *The Headaches.*

Headaches in Children and Adolescents

Migraine-type headaches can occur in children as young as three years old. They usually hold their foreheads and say it hurts, may get sick, and then go sleep. When they wake up, they feel refreshed, and their headaches are gone. What happens further depends to a large degree on the history of headaches in the family. There is also some correlation between severities of headaches in parents

2000 Lippincot Williams and Wilkins Philadelphia Pennsylvania (PA) and children. Most children get an occasional headache and respond to a nap. Some of them start getting headaches three to four times a month or even more by the time they are six to eight years of age. They may need pain pills, such as acetaminophen (Tylenol). If Tylenol doesn't help, 200mg of Motrin (or Advil) can be tried. I have used 25mg of sumatriptan (Imitrex) in children as young as six years old. By the time these children reach puberty, the majority of boys quit having headaches. On the contrary, half the girls continue to have headaches, which can become more severe and more frequent. Some of the girls develop menstrual migraines. Children rarely get tension-type headaches. After puberty, a small number of young ladies can develop tension-type headaches. Children who get repeat headaches should get a CAT scan or an MRI. It is also worth noting that children with migraines rarely get auras.

Treatment

As mentioned above, Tylenol and ibuprofen should be tried first. Next, one can use 25mg to 50mg of sumatriptan (Imitrex), 2.5mg of naratriptan, or 2.5mg to 5mg of zolmitriptan. Dihydroergotamine (DHE) 0.5mg to 1 mg nasal spray can also be tried. One should avoid narcotics or Fiorinal, which contains barbiturates.

Prophylactic Treatment

Some children need preventive treatment if headaches are frequent and severe.

Cyproheptidine (Periactin)

This is an anti-allergy medicine with anti-5HT properties. Its dose is 4mg to 12mg a day in divided doses. It works in 50 percent of patients. It causes sleepiness, dry mouth, and weight gain. It is not used very often these days.

Beta-Blockers

Propranolol **(Inderal)**

It is safe and easily tolerated and works in about 65 percent of patients. It should not be prescribed if there is a history of asthma. To start with, the patient can be given 20mg a day and can be increased up to 80mg a day.

Calcium Channel Blockers

Verapamil **(Calan)**

The patient can be started at 40mg and can go up to 160mg a day, which is fairly effective.

Antidepressants

Amitriptyline **(Elavil)**

Patients as young as eight years old can be given this medication. The dose can be 10mg to 30mg at bedtime.

Protriptyline **(Vivactil)**

This medication should be given in the morning at a dose of 10mg to 20mg a day. This medication works in more than 50 percent of patients.

Anticonvulsants

Valproic Acid **(Depakote)**

Patients can be given 250mg to 750mg a day. This medication has worked in over 70 percent of cases. It rarely causes liver problems, but blood work should be done periodically.

Diet

Children with frequent migraines should give up pizza, chocolate, and cola drinks. If patients follow this even for six months, headaches do improve. After the headaches improve, patients can eat and drink these foods occasionally, one at a time, to see which foods or drinks cause headaches.

CHAPTER 14

Other Headaches

Headaches Associated with Sexual Activity

This is usually a dull, acute pain in the head and neck that intensifies as sexual excitement increases. This is far more common in men than in women. Both intercourse and masturbation cause headache, which is mild but intensifies by the time of coitus. Use of Cafergot or Indocin 30mg thirty minutes before the activity can sometimes avoid this kind of pain.

Cough Headaches

These can be prevented as well by taking Indocin 25–50mg thirty minutes beforehand.

Headaches Associated with Vascular Disease such as Migraine and Stroke

Stroke under the age of fifty is not too uncommon in patients with migraines. About 9 percent of the migraine populations have strokes. The diagnosis of acute venous thrombosis is characterized by headache and increased pressure in the eye (papilledema). Headaches, seizures, focal deficit (loss of function of some part of the body), coma, and sometimes death occur with stroke associated with migraines. A CAT scan of the brain or magnetic resonance tomography is quite helpful in making this diagnosis.

Treatment should be started as soon as possible. Anticonvulsants, intravenous heparin (blood thinners), and measures to decrease intracranial pressure should be used. Antibiotics, if there is an infection, as well as steroids should be used if necessary. Painkillers including opiates can be used. The prognosis seems to be better than before; however, the death rate is still 25 percent.

Thunderclap Headaches

This is the sudden onset of severe headaches that reach a maximum intensity in one minute or so. There is no other severe acute onset of headaches, although migraines can sometimes present in this manner. It also occurs due to a rupture of intracranial aneurysms.

Carotid Artery Pain

Carotidynia is severe pain in a carotid artery that sometimes occurs on both sides. It is a unilateral pain and sometimes associated with swelling. The causes include blocking of a carotid artery, fibromuscular dysplasia (beadlike thickening of the blood vessels), carotid dissection (tear in the artery with associated blockage of the artery), giant cell arthritis (inflammation of the artery), carotid body tumors, and migraine disease.

Cervical and cerebral artery dissections are an important part of ischemic strokes. In terms of classical tissue disease, arterial hypertension and migraine are the underlying causes. Head pain is really the only sign of dissection. Unilateral headache and neck pain in a patient presenting with anterior cerebral artery attacks is a common example.

Chronic Paroxysmal Hemicrania

This is characterized by pain associated with symptoms and signs of cluster headaches, but it is shorter lasting. It usually responds to indomethacin. This type of headache is increasing in frequency, especially in Norway, the Czech Republic, Denmark, Italy, France, Mexico, the United Kingdom, Canada, Sweden, Australia, Germany, Poland, India, Spain, Brazil, South Africa, and New Zealand.

Chronic paroxysmal hemicrania is far more common in women. The mean age of onset is thirty-four years. Once again, Indocin (indomethacin) is the preferred drug for treatment.

Clinical features
At least forty attacks a day
Attacks are more common on one side than the other
Redness of conjunctiva
Stuffiness of nose
Swelling of eyelids

Nighttime Attacks
Attacks vary from thirty to ninety-five year of age; they are more commonly seen in women. They can last as long as 4,500 to 10,524 hours.

Treatment
Indocin is a wonder drug for this condition. Sometimes, the dose needs to be increased. The usual dose of Indocin is 25mg two times a day, but it may have to be increased to 50mg three or four times a day. Besides Indocin, there is verapamil, aspirin, piroxicam (Feldene), amitriptyline, lithium, and Tegretol.

Idiopathic Stabbing Headaches
These are ice pick–like pain, jabs, and jolts associated with pain in the eye. These are described as stabs of pain in the head that occur spontaneously in the absence of organic disease or any kind of abnormality of the cranial nerves.

Clinical profile
Pain is localized in the head, usually in the frontotemporal as well as parietal areas.

Pain is stabbing, lasting for a few seconds.
The periodicity varies from hours to days.

Cold-Stimulation Headaches

These are properly called ice-cream headaches and also cold-stimulation headaches. The essential factor is exposure to cold, ice, and anything at subzero temperatures.

> It is characterized by the presence of cold stimulus.
> It lasts for four to six minutes.
> Pain is in the middle of the forehead.
> In patients with migraines, the pain affects the usual area of migraines.

Holding on to the throat and then swallowing can relieve the headache in some patients.

Benign Cough Headaches

These headaches, brought on by coughing, occur on both sides of the head and last for about a month. They can be avoided by avoiding coughing. The majority of patients are male (92 percent). The average age is fifty-five years. Treatment is Indocin 50mg three times a day; Inderal and ergotamine can also be effective. Spinal tap can help some of these headaches.

Benign Exertional Headaches

This category includes any kind of headache brought on by physical activity or exercise.

Clinical profile

It is brought on by any kind of exercise.
It usually affects both sides of the head.

It can last for ten to forty-five minutes.

Working in hot weather or high altitudes is more likely to bring on such a headache.

Weight lifting and swimming can cause fairly sudden headache.

Treatment

Taking Indocin 50–150mg or ergotamine 1 mg can often prevent these headaches. Motrin or other anti-inflammatory agents can also be useful.

Clinical profile

Dull ache in the head and neck that intensifies as sexual activity increases

Sudden and severe headache occurring at orgasm

Posterior headache resembles that of lower spinal fluid pressure, and the pressure develops at the time of coitus

Treatment

Ergotamine 1–2mg thirty minutes before sexual activity; Indocin 50–150mg thirty minutes before sexual activity; Diltiazem (calcium channel blocker) 60mg three times a day; or Inderal 40–200mg taken daily with a dose thirty minutes before sexual activity.

Hemicrania Continua

This is a one-sided daily headache that is new and responds to Indocin. It usually lasts for one month. The severity is moderate. It is also associated with the following:

Swelling of eyelids
Drooping of eyelids
Watering of the eyes
Redness of the eyes
Watering of the nose
Redness of the eyes and congestion of the nose

Headaches Associated with Vascular Diseases

Migraine Headaches and Strokes

About 8 percent of the populations with migraines have strokes. Patients are usually below the age of fifty years. In women, strokes usually occur below the age of forty-four years. The risk in women is higher if they use oral contraceptives and smoke.

Migrainous Cerebral Infarction

These patients usually have migraines with auras. The presence of ischemic infarctions is substantiated by MRI and angiography.

Migraines can produce strokes in many ways:

Stroke may arise as a result of a migraine attack.

Stroke may result from existence of migraines.

Both migraine and stroke with subcortical (below the surface of the outer layer of the brain) stroke or infarctions occur.

Headaches and Stroke Syndromes

Headaches occur with ischemic strokes (infarction of the brain caused by poor circulation to a territory of the brain or sudden onset intracerebral bleeding). This can also produce sudden changes in the level of consciousness.

Subarachnoid Hemorrhage

This is also acute in onset with changes in level of consciousness and evidence of blood on CT scan or angiography. (Angiography is done by the insertion of a catheter in the groin and injecting a dye, which usually confirms the diagnosis.) Recently, magnetic resonance angiography has gained popularity because it requires a very small amount of dye.

Aneurysms (Swelling on a Weakened Wall)

This is the most common cause of a subarachnoid bleed, but it can occur from an arteriovenous malformation and a tendency to have a bleeding problem.

Headaches Associated with Vascular Procedures

Carotid Endarterectomy (Opening the Carotid Artery to Remove a Clot)

Sometimes, the stroke does not occur right away, but after a few days, there is a sudden onset of pain on the side of the carotid artery, which points to the fact that something like that must have happened. The medications that can be used are Fiorinal and Indocin.

Angiitis of the Central Nervous System

Angiitis means inflammation, which occurs in various forms and distributions. Primary angiitis of the central nervous system has many names. Headaches are a symptom in 58 percent of patients. Besides headaches, symptoms include incoordination, focal neurological deficit, seizures, changes in mental status, and changes in level of consciousness. Treatments include verapamil (calcium channel blocker), Depakote, and newer anticonvulsants such as topiramate, gabapentin, or Lamictal, or a small dose of aspirin could be used. Beta-blockers such as Inderal and others should not be used.

Giant Cell Arthritis (Temporal Arthritis)

Temporal arthritis is a disease that usually starts late in life, usually about the age of sixty years. There is inflammation of the arteries. Headaches are extremely common. There can also be intermittent pain in the jaw, known as claudication of the jaw. Loss of vision is fairly common. There is stiffness of the shoulders and arms. Sometimes, hips have stiffness as well. Its incidence is described to be four per hundred thousand.

The pathology reveals skipped areas of inflammation with multiple kinds of abnormal cells. The blood vessels are narrow. In addition to the symptoms described above, there are temporal headaches, headaches located on the sides of the head, which can be one side or both sides; neck, ear, and throat pain; scalp tenderness; and facial, eye, and gum pain.

Regarding the blood test (sed rate), if a tube is filled with blood, the rate at which the blood cells settle down determines the sed rate. This test is usually 60 percent diagnostic. Biopsy of the temporal artery is sometimes the only way to confirm diagnosis. Signs of tender temporal artery are suggestive of this condition.

Treatment
Initially, a high dose of prednisone for two to three months is the best thing to do. Later on, one of the anticancer drugs (methotrexate) can be added, so the dose of prednisone can be decreased. As time progresses, the intensity of the disease becomes less virulent (benign). In about two years, this disease has a tendency to almost die down.

Systemic Lupus Erythematosus (SLE)
This is an autoimmune disease that in some ways resembles multiple sclerosis. Headaches can be off and on but can last for a long time. Lupus can occur at any age. It is more common in women. Headaches are present in about 40 percent of patients.

Criteria for SLE

Red rash on the cheeks
Photosensitivity
Pleural effusion or pericarditis (inflammation of the covering of the lungs or the heart)
Arthritis
Kidney disease

Seizures or psychosis
Anemia due to breakdown of red blood cells
Antinuclear antibodies are usually elevated
Headaches lasting for four to eight months
Off-and-on inflammation of the arteries
SE cells found in 70 percent of patients; sed rate usually elevated

Treatment

Use of anticancer drugs such as azathioprine and cyclophosphamide are very useful. Steroids can be used and sometimes plasmapheresis as well. The patient's life can be prolonged to almost close to normal.

Headache Associated with Intracranial Infection

Headaches occur at the onset of intracranial infection and go away after successful treatment of the infection.

Clinical profile

Severe headache
Confusion
Neck stiffness
Stupor
Coma and seizures

Sarcoidosis

This is a noninfectious condition with granulomas (nonmalignant or benign tumors that are not infective either). These tumors are seen in the lungs, brain, eyes, skin, and lymph nodes. Involvement of the brain occurs in about 8 percent of patients. Some patients develop weakness on one or both sides of the face. Some patients also develop increased pressure in the head associated with diffuse headaches, nausea, vomiting, and changes in level of consciousness.

Treatment

Prednisone (steroids) starting with a high dose and then slowly tapering or decreasing the dose is the best way to treat these headaches. The treatment can be repeated if necessary.

Intracranial Tumors

Headaches start at the beginning of a brain tumor in 18 percent of patients. As time goes on, the headache increases to 55 percent of patients. The headaches usually occur on the side of the tumor but can occur on both sides in some instances. In some patients with metastatic tumors (tumors that spread from other places such as lungs, kidney, breast, etc.), the headache may have characteristics of a tension-type headache or a migraine-type headache.

Management is Lasix (furosemide) 40–160mg a day and can be gradually increased to 2gram a day if necessary. Some patients require an intracranial peritoneal shunt, which means draining the fluid from the brain into the abdomen. A lumboperitoneal shunt is needed in some patients; this requires putting a shunt between the lumbar spine and into the abdomen. Finally, radiation treatment or chemotherapy may be needed later. Diamox (water pill) is started in two divided doses to begin with and increased to 2gram a day.

Subarachnoid Hemorrhage

The headache due to a subarachnoid bleed (bleeding between the second layer of the covering the arachnoids and pia layers) occurs almost instantaneously. It is usually severe but sometimes can be mild to moderate. There is usually stiffness of the neck, nausea, vomiting, sensitivity to light, and changes in level of consciousness. The most common cause is aneurysms (ballooning of blood vessels that are weak to begin with and rupture under pressure). The other causes of subarachnoid bleeds include a rupture of an arteriovenous malformation, head trauma, and, rarely, certain brain tumors.

The diagnosis is made by computed axial tomography (CAT) scan and is confirmed by spinal tap, which reveals increased pressure and a few red cells in the spinal fluid as well as yellow discoloration of the spinal fluid known as xanthochromia.

Treatment depends on the condition of the patient. For patients who are almost comatose, no surgery is usually contemplated. The calcium channel blocker Nimotop (nimodipine), 30mg four times a day, can be used. This, however, is useful only in mild to moderate cases. For less severe patients, an angiogram is warranted. This shows the exact location of the aneurysm. Most surgeons prefer to wait for seven to ten days before surgery is considered. In patients who are totally alert, surgery can be done in two to three days. The surgery consists of tying the neck of the aneurysm. A flexible coil is injected into the aneurysm, which prevents further bleeding.

General measures such as intravenous fluids to decrease intracranial pressure and anticonvulsants are necessary. If there is significant swelling of the brain, use of steroids for a short period is warranted.

Headaches Associated with Diseases of the Ears, Nose, and Throat

This is a rather common condition. There are two parts to this condition. The first is an allergic condition with chronic stuffiness of the nose; this very rarely causes a significant headache. Diseases of the sinuses do cause significant headaches. Most of the time, there is infection in the sinuses, most likely bacterial but sometimes fungal. The symptoms develop on the location of the sinus that is involved—if the infection is in the frontal sinuses, the front part of the head is affected, but the headache can radiate backward. If only one side of the frontal sinuses is involved, the pain is usually on that side. If the infection is in the sphenoid sinus, the pain is deep and to some degree in the frontal area as well. The third sinus is the ethmoid sinus, which gets infected rather uncommonly; however, if it does get infected, the pain is behind the nose.

It is absolutely necessary to get a CAT scan of the sinuses without intravenous contrast. This shows clearly the location and extent of the infection. Some patients will get repeated sinus infections, the most common cause being a polyp or a cyst, which blocks the area and makes the infection possible.

If there is no cyst or polyp on the CAT scan, the treatment is a course of antibiotics for a period of three to four weeks. An intranasal spray of steroids usually helps as well. Polyps, if present, should be surgically removed.

Temporomandibular Joint Disorder (TMJ)

Clinical profile

Pain of the jaw brought on by chewing
Noise during jaw movement
Pain on pressure of the joint
Decrease of movement

Treatment
The medications that can be used are antiarthritis medications (nonsteroidal anti-inflammatory agents) or injection of steroids, pain medications, muscle relaxants, antidepressants, and anticonvulsants. Physical therapy, ultrasound, moist heat, and muscle-strengthening exercises may also be in order.

CHAPTER 15
Trigeminal Neuralgia

Trigeminal neuralgia is an acute, painful condition affecting one of the three divisions of the trigeminal nerve, which supplies sensation to one side of the face. The first division affects the frontal area, the second division affects the cheeks, and the third division affects the mandible. Trigeminal neuralgia is a condition that occurs usually after the age of fifty or even later. The condition is confined to only one side and then to only one division at a time. Sometimes much later during the course of the disease, it can spread to both sides.

The pain is excruciating and feels like electric shock–like pain. It usually lasts for less than thirty seconds and rarely beyond sixty seconds. There can be hundreds of such attacks in a twenty-four-hour period. The pain can last for three to six months and then subsides. In terms of resemblance to headaches, only when the pain is in the frontal division is the character of pain sometimes difficult to differentiate between migraine and trigeminal neuralgia.

On examination, there is hyperesthesia (increased sensation with touch and pinprick in the affected area). There are no diagnostic studies to arrive at a diagnosis. If the pain does not go away after trying two or three medications, MRI is warranted to make sure there is no tumor, infection, or arteriovenous malformation.

The first line of treatment is medications. Anticonvulsants are the most effective. Tegretol and Neurontin are both equally effective. Dilantin and Lioresal are in the next order of drugs.

Drug	Dose (mg a day)
Tegretol	600
Neurontin	1,200–2,400
Dilantin	300
Lioresal	30

If medicine does not work at all, there are a couple of surgical procedures that are fairly effective. Some of the lesser procedures are injections in the ganglions with alcohol or glycerol; partial destruction of the ganglion with radiofrequency lesions; and radiosurgery by Gamma knife. Sometimes there is a loop of blood vessels pressing over the trigeminal nerve; if that is removed, the face pain goes away.

Postherpetic Neuralgia

This is an infection caused by herpes zoster. Pain occurs in the frontal area on one side. It is a rather severe, painful condition. If the pain is not treated, it lasts for about ten weeks or so. Pain can be relieved in ninety-six hours after steroid treatment.

Postherpetic neuralgia develops after three to four years. This pain is different as it is burning, stabbing pain with some itching.

Oral steroids, oral antiviral agents (Acyclovir, Fanciclovir), amitriptyline (Elavil), capsaicin (applied locally), and local anesthetics can all be effective treatments.

Postherpetic neuralgia occurs in patients who have had chicken pox during childhood. The virus sits in the trigeminal ganglia for years, and some patients in their old age develop herpes zoster.

CHAPTER 16

Headaches from Street Drugs

- There are many chemicals and drugs that cause headaches.
- Monosodium glutamate (MSG) is used quite liberally in Asian foods. -In addition to severe headaches, there is tightness of the chest and abdominal discomfort.
- Carbon monoxide causes headaches, nausea, vomiting, blurred vision, confusion, and finally coma and death.
- Alcohol headaches occur in susceptible patients.
- Nitrates and nitrites are present in hot dogs and people who handle nitroglycerin. They usually get headaches only. Nitroglycerin workers in factories tend to get these headaches.
- Food additives
    Aspartame—those who use excessive amounts tend to get headaches. Children, in addition, get hyperactivity.
    Tyramine is present in chocolate and cheese. They tend to produce migraine-type headaches.
    Phenylethylamine is present in chocolate and cocoa and presents migraine-like headaches.

- Street drugs
  Chronic repeat use of cocaine can cause severe headache, confusion, stroke-like symptoms, heart attacks, loss of vision, and seizures.
- Crack cocaine causes severe headaches and stroke.
- Marijuana causes mild and both-sided headaches, facial pain, and muscle spasms.

Headaches from Chronic Use of Drugs (Chronic Use of Medications)

Criteria of Diagnosis
Headaches occur after daily use of four months. These headaches are chronic, coming on fifteen to twenty times a month. The headaches disappear once the drug is stopped for four to five weeks.

Ergotamine-Induced Headache
This occurs due to daily use of 1 mg oral dose or 2mg rectal dose. The headache is pulsating and on both sides of the head. Ergotamine withdrawal is needed for four to six weeks for headaches to go away.

Drugs Taken by Patients with Drug-Induced Headaches

Valium
Xanax
Ativan
Opiates
Codeine

Simple analgesics
Salicylates (aspirin)
Phenothiazines
Indomethacin
Dihydroergotamine
Ergotamine
Barbiturates
Caffeine

Headaches in Psychiatric Diseases

Headaches in the group of psychiatric diseases are not very common. Out of the group, they are most common in depression, and then, in decreasing order, in anxiety, hysteria, and schizophrenia. No specific treatment is required for headaches in particular.

Drug Abuse and Headaches

About 13 percent of headaches in the population occur due to overuse of drugs.

Drugs commonly used are as follows:

Benzodiazepines
Valium
Lithium
·Ativan
Clonazepam
Xanax
Dalmane
Restoril
Halcion
Ultram
Stadol
Darvon

Methadone
Codeine
Oxycodone
Hydrocodone
Duragesic
Oxymorphone

Headache Medications (Commonly Used)

Ergotamine tartrate
Triptans

Mixed analgesics

- Vicodin
- Esgic Plus
- Esgic
- Fiorinal
- Vicodin ES
- Fiorinal with codeine

Drugs should be gradually withdrawn so patients do not get withdrawal symptoms. This may take three to four weeks. Then the medicines that are absolutely essential could be reintroduced. If the patient takes many narcotics, an attempt should be made to change to lesser pain medications. Similarly, pain pills, triptans, and others should be introduced with caution.

Association of Headaches with Sleep

Sleep disorders and headaches, especially migraines, are common phenomena. It is a well-known fact that too much sleep, especially on weekends, makes people get headaches. To a lesser degree, too little sleep can also cause headaches. If someone is getting a headache and takes a nap, the headache usually gets better. Many other times, if someone decides to take a nap, he or she wakes up with a headache.

Patients with cluster headaches usually get clusters 90 to 120 minutes after sleeping and then early in the morning, such as 4:00 a.m. Most patients with migraines also usually wake up with headaches.

Sometimes, unpleasant dreams, including having a migraine during the dream state, can cause one to wake up with a migraine headache.

Hypnic Headaches

Hypnic headaches are a subtype of cluster-type headaches that occur during sleep.

CHAPTER 17

Migraine Headaches in Pregnancy

In most women with a history of migraines, these headaches get worse during the first three to four months of pregnancy. Headaches get much better during the second and third trimesters of pregnancy. There are some women who continue to get headaches until the baby is delivered.

Treatment is very tricky. Most medications have the possibility of producing birth defects. The safest thing is to start with Tylenol. If that does not work, one should consider biofeedback, which can provide good results in some patients. After that, and if using narcotics, one can try Tylenol with codeine. Codeine has a tendency to cause nausea and stomach irritation. If that does not work, one needs to use a meperidine (Demerol) 50–100mg every six to eight hours. Some women who cannot eat and have bad headaches need hospital admission to be given IV fluids and IV Demerol. There is no 100 percent prophylactic medicine that is safe. As a last resort, one can try a beta-blocker like Inderal or an antidepressant medicine like amitriptyline. None of the triptans are safe to use.

Some of the newer treatments are as follows:

- Botulism injections for chronic migraines. Thirty-one sites in the head and neck are chosen with a maximum dose of 195 units. Specific headache reduction usually takes place. The incidence of infection by these injections is only 5 percent.
- Increased risk of cerebrovascular and cardiovascular disease in patients with a history of migraines and strokes is 2 percent of migraines, 1.2 percent in migraines with aura, and 1 percent without aura.
- Occipital nerve stimulation shows some promise in refractory migraine cases. This consists of stimulating the back part of the head with the nerve stimulator a couple times a week for several weeks.
- Transcranial magnetic stimulation, which is done through the use of magnets, can improve headaches.
- Doxycycline can be effective in getting rid of daily headaches.
- A combination of Viatral, magnesium, and coenzyme Q_{10}.
- Electrical stimulation behind the ear.
- Dural stimulation for chronic headaches is a direct stimulation through a hole in the skull, done many times a week for many weeks.
- Antioxidants (ten capsules per day) of 120mg pink bark extract, 60mg of vitamin C, and 20 IU of vitamin E improved nine out of eleven patients with chronic migraines.[4]

Patent foramen Ovule

- Repair of the patent foramen ovule can improve headaches after surgical repair of the defect. Blood returning from the body moves through the head from the right atrium to the right ventricle, and this is sent to the lungs to have carbon dioxide removed; oxygen passes from the left atrium into the left ventricle through the rest of the body through the

---

4 Stephen Silberstein, Richard Lipton, and Donald Dalessio, eds., *Wolff's Headache and Other Head Pain.*

aorta. The foramen ovule is a flap between the left atrium and right atrium. This flap remains open because of equal pressure in both the left and right atria. At birth, pressure in the left atrium rises quickly, which closes the flap, which eventually gets permanently shut with further development of scar tissue. For unknown reasons, the flap remains open in 25 percent of patients. In patients with patent foramen ovule, very little blood passes from the left to the right ventricle.

During hard coughing or sneezing, pressure on the right side can increase, and the flap opens and passes blood from the right to the left side. Physicians have noted for a long time that leg clots can pass to the left side of the heart, causing strokes. When such patients have surgery to close the flap, strokes stop. Patients also notice that headaches stop as well.

Prevention of cluster headaches

Intranasal civamide 100mg a day
Suboccipital steroid injection
Melatonin 10mg a day
Sumatriptan or zolmitriptan as a nasal spray
Occipital nerve stimulation for chronic cluster headaches
Intravenous aspirin (lysine and acetylsalicylate) in the patient
    management of headaches

Complex Regional Pain Syndrome (Reflex Sympathetic Dystrophy)

This is a rather complex pain syndrome without a well-known cause that attacks one extremity, more so part of the limb away from the body. There are no diagnostic or blood tests for this disease. If the pain lasts too long for the injury or takes a long time to worsen, this condition is usually considered.

There are no good treatments. The applicative measures are pain, autonomic changes such as bluish discoloration of the arms and legs, and swelling. These symptoms are important in making the diagnosis.

Treatment

Treatment involves relaxation, biofeedback and stress management, and use of drugs for pain, neuropathic pain in particular. Nonsteroidal anti-inflammatory drugs, opiates, and antidepressants all work to some degree, but not every patient responds the same way. Alpha-adrenergic blockers (prazosin or doxazosin) can be used. Membrane stabilizers can be used; these fall in the category of anticonvulsants or antiepileptic drugs. Corticosteroids, such as prednisone or Decadron, can be used, as well as capsaicin, which is used more as a local or topical agent.

Airplane Headaches

These occur mostly in men in the front and side of the head during the time of descent and last for twenty to thirty minutes. Pain is moderate to severe but not throbbing and not associated with any other symptoms. It can be treated by taking one of the nonsteroidal anti-inflammatory drugs half an hour before descent. Change in cabin pressure may have something to do with it. These patients should have clinical and radiological studies of their sinuses, as well as the pharynx and larynx (back part of the throat and the breathing tube) because they can cause severe headaches. This condition has been described by Schoenen and colleagues in *Neurology*.[5] Other studies are needed because Schoenen et al.'s sample was rather small.

Carbon Dioxide (CO_2) Accumulation Headache

Some patients who sleep with their faces and heads covered can get headaches when they wake up. Sleeping in a somewhat cool room without covers on their faces would help this situation.

---

5 J. Schoenen, B. Vandermissen, S. Jeangette, et al., "Migraine Prevention with a Supraorbital Transcutaneous Stimulator: A Randomized Controlled Trial," *Neurology* 80, no. 8 (2013): 697–704.

New Treatment (Electrical Stimulation)

Stimulation of the sphenopalatine ganglion would obtain relief and less frequent attacks. The nerve fibers of this ganglion are located in the back part of the nose as well as the throat. A total of twenty-eight patients were studied by Schoenen et al. Acute response occurred in 25 percent of patients, and in 50 percent of the patients, there was a frequent reduction in the pain. Thirty-two percent of patients did not respond at all. Further research would need to be done to help evaluate the use of this procedure.

CHAPTER 18

Conclusion

After reading this book, you will realize that some of the more common causes of primary headaches, such as migraine headaches, tension headaches, and cluster headaches, have been written about in a fair degree of detail. I also attempted to touch on many of the uncommon headaches to make this book a complete compendium.

The idea of going through the book is to get through as many causes of headaches as possible. The book was not written so that the reader can make a self-diagnosis. Rather, it was written to arm the reader with knowledge for a visit to the physician so that he or she can ask pertinent and pointed questions to lead to a diagnosis, tests, treatment, and so forth. For example, if the physician is quick and rushes through an appointment, the reader, after reading this book, should realize that it may be necessary to get a CAT scan or an MRI to make sure there are no other causes of headaches besides migraines. One pertinent example is if someone has double vision, dizziness, and weakness on one side; these problems are probably indicative of something more than migraines.

I hope you enjoyed reading the book as much as I enjoyed writing it. I also hope you found the reading easy and useful.

www.ingramcontent.com/pod-product-compliance
Lightning Source LLC
Chambersburg PA
CBHW070924290526
45795CB00001B/415